CW01370235

KAMA SUTRA SEX POSITIONS

DISCOVER A SURPRISINGLY NEW WAY TO EXPERIENCE SEXUALITY. IMPROVE YOUR LOVEMAKING, INCREASE INTIMACY, AND REACH EXTRAORDINARY ORGASMS

Amanda Shein

TABLE OF CONTENTS:

INTRODUCTION 5
KAMA SUTRA SEX POSITIONS 9
KAMA SUTRA EROTIC MASSAGE 19
HOW TO PREPARE THE BODY 24
EMBRACES 30
LOVE AND THE KAMA SUTRA 39
SACRED SEXUAL ROLE OF WOMEN 51
PRACTICING LOVE MAKING FOR A HEALTHY BODY AND MIND 62
KAMA SUTRA AND COURTESANS 72
KISSING TECHNIQUES: THE KAMA SUTRA'S SUBTLE FORMS OF SENSUALITY. 82
HOW TO REACH ECSTASY IN 10 DIFFERENCE POSITION 89
STEP-BY-STEP POSITIONS FOR THE BEGINNER 98
CONCLUSION 107

Introduction

It is unlikely that you have never heard of the Kama Sutra before, but you may be unfamiliar with what exactly it is. Some may think of it as simply a book of sex positions, while others may know a bit more of the history and how it came to be. This chapter will look at the history behind the Kama Sutra, discussing the literal meaning of the words, as well as what it teaches us, and how it is meant to be used. Since the Kama Sutra originated in India, there are also many terms and words used throughout that you may not be familiar with, so we will make sure to breakdown some of the most commonly seen ones and provide their definitions.

With such a rich history behind it, there is so much to learn about the Kama Sutra. It is an expansive work of literature that was created to be more than just a guide on different ways in which you can have sex. Instead, it permeates all aspects of life and brings together both sexual and non-sexual ways in which you interact with a lover, a partner, or a spouse. But what exactly does "Kama Sutra" mean?

Meaning Behind the Name

The word Kama is one that means pleasure but can also be translated as desire or longing. There is a sexual connotation associated with the word, meaning it is more to do with sexual pleasure and desire than with the pleasures of life or desire for material goods, but that doesn't mean that the Kama Sutra as a whole is limited to only sexual pleasure. Sutra, on the other hand, translates to verse or scripture. When you put these words together, you get the translation of "Scripture of Pleasure", but there are many variations on how you can literally translate this.

Delving deeper into the meaning behind the name, the pleasure that is Kama is one that is of all five senses, and this is very important. While many thinks of the Kama Sutra as a sex book, it is actually a book that focuses on pleasing all of the senses and is meant to be a guide on how to live a good life and enjoy yourself. From the physical enjoyment of sex to the pleasure that is derived from being in love, the Kama Sutra is filled with different verses that cover a wide range of different activities and pleasures.

While we did mention that Kama often has a sexual connotation, like with all translations there are different meanings depending on how it is being used. Kama can also be used when referencing love or affection, and in this sense, it is used in a non-sexual way. This is why the Kama Sutra needs to be viewed as a whole, since it was not intended to simply be a sexual book, but more so an erotic manual on life.

We know that the Kama Sutra extends beyond just the physical pleasures, as the book touches on the four different virtues of life. Those four are:

- Dharma – How to live a virtuous life

- Kama – How to enjoy the pleasures of the senses
- Moksha – How to be liberated from the cycle of reincarnation
- Artha – How to gain material wealth

These four virtues are tenants of Hinduism, which is applicable since the Kama Sutra originates in India where Hinduism is one of the predominant religions. This historical context allows us to understand the book better, as we need to approach it from the mindset of the author, who would have most likely been a practicing Hindu. The author saw sexual pleasure as one of the main virtues of life, and it was both a necessary and spiritual pursuit that was important both from a non-sexual and sexual avenue. These virtues are almost instructions on how a person should live in order to be fulfilled both in this life as well as in the afterlife. Regardless of what your personal religion is, all the points are still applicable, as basic human nature dictates that we are all attempting to be the best version of ourselves and to accomplish everything we set out to gain.

Some other words that you may encounter within the Kama Sutra, and their translations, are:

- Devi – Goddess
- Gandharva – A form of marriage in which everyone is consenting to it
- Lingam – Penis
- Nayika – A woman who is desired by someone
- Prahanana – Striking or slapping someone during sex
- Raja – King
- Shlokas – Messages from above that are used to end every chapter of the Kama Sutra

- Vatsala – A married woman who has children
- Vikrant – A brave and beloved man
- Yoni – Vagina

Within this book, we will try and use as much of the original language as possible, so having a glossary of terms will be beneficial. With that said, however, there will always be translations available throughout so that you can follow along with ease.

So why does the literal meaning of the name even matter?

Well, understanding what an author is trying to convey is important as it allows us to enter the book and adjust our personal views so that we do not bring in our biases and preconceived notions. If you come into the Kama Sutra thinking it should only include some sex positions and nothing more, then you miss out on the richness that is contained within. Likewise, if you ignore the historical significance behind the text, you fail to grasp many of the concepts located within. In order to gain as much as you can from the Kama Sutra, you need to know what the author intended with it, and why they felt the need to create this work of literature.

Kama Sutra Sex Positions

The Kama Sutra boasts many different positions a couple can try during lovemaking. These range from being complex muscle movements to soft, sexy postures, which means there is something to accommodate every one of widely varying body types and physical capabilities.

The wide variety of poses listed in the Kama Sutra ensures that everyone is going to find something they are intrigued by and want to try. There are poses that include lying down, standing up, sitting, man on top, woman on top, facing one another and the list goes on and on.

From a technical standpoint, sex is a strange and peculiar act with two people engaged in positions that seem to defy gravitational law, breathing heavily, and moving rapidly as bodily fluids are exchanged between them. This aside, sex can be a fatiguing and somewhat unpleasant act just as equally as it can be a pleasurable, satisfying, and beneficial experience. The more creative you get and the more you work to create a positive atmosphere in bed, the better you will feel and the more capable you will be at communicating positive feelings towards your partner.

The following is a listing of some of the sexual positions described in the Kama Sutra:

Of the lying down positions, the "**widely open position**" is performed when the woman lowers her head back and raises her middle parts awaiting penetration from the man.

The "**yawning position**" is when a woman raises her thighs and keeps them wide apart to engage in congress.

When both the male and female stretch their legs out over each other, this is called the "**clasping position**", and once the embrace has begun in this position and the woman presses her lover with her thighs, it is the "**pressing position.**"

The "**rising position**" is achieved when the woman raises both of her thighs straight up, and when only one of her legs remains stretched out, it is called the "**half pressed position.**"

The "**erotic V**" is a position that requires some flexibility. The woman wraps her arms around his neck while sitting on a table edge with her legs up and her bottom at the edge of the table. The man stands directly in front of her and bends his legs if necessary, to achieve the best entry point.

The "**splitting bamboo**" is when the woman places her leg over her lover's shoulder, then stretches out her other leg and places this upon his shoulder and continues to do so alternately.

The "**catherine wheel**" is a position in which the man and the woman sit facing each other and the woman wraps her legs around the man's waist until he penetrates her. To support herself, the woman leans back with her hands up off the bed.

The "**x rated**" is a position where the male partner lays face up on the bed, and the female partner straddles her partner with her back to his face. She lowers her hips for penetration and after penetration, she lowers her upper body between his legs and extends her own legs out straight. His and her legs create the letter x. She slides her body forward and backward, up and down.

The "**thigh master**" is a position in which the male lies down on his back, but instead of stretching his legs in the outward direction, he bends the legs at the knees. With her back facing the partner, the female straddles him. After that, she lowers onto his penis and places her knees on the bed. Her right knee is on the outside of his right thigh, and her left knee is placed between his legs on the bed.

The "**star**" is a position in which the female lies down on her back with one of the legs outstretched and the other leg bent at her knee. While the female is in this position, her outstretched leg is straddled by the male partner who gently nudges one of his knees under his partner's bottom. Then, he leans back, holding his body weight on his arms placed behind him. The male controls penetration, but the female is free to get pleasure from this.

The "**doggy style**" is a position in which the female is on her hands and knees with her legs spread wide to let her partner do the process of penetration from behind. The male partner kneels down and enters from behind while grabbing on to her hips or thighs. The female keeps shifting her weight forward and backward as required during the process to attain maximum pleasure. Both partners have the ability to control the rhythm, speed and depth of penetration during doggy style sex.

The "**curled angel**" is a position in which both the male and female lie on their sides while the male remains embraced to the back side of the female. The female draws her legs towards her chest which allows for easy penetration from behind. This position can also be used during pregnancy with the exception that the female's legs will not rest that close to her chest. The male can either stretch his legs out straight or spoon them into his partner's legs depending upon the comfort level of both the partners.

The "**hound**" is a position in which the female gets on all fours, but her upper body weight is rested on the forearms instead of the hands. Her thighs are pressed together to make easy for the male partner to place one of his knees on the outside of each of her legs. He penetrates from the rear side and then bends his upper body over her bottom. He can also hold on to her body or breasts while controlling penetration and rhythm during the process.

The "**visitor**" is a position which the male and female stand facing each other with her arms wrapped around his back and his hands holding on to her hips and bottom. After using his penis to stimulate her, he enters from the front. She can lift her leg slightly to the outside of his thighs to ease penetration.

The "**standing wheelbarrow**" is a position in which the female starts the position with knees and hands on the floor in Doggy Style. Her partner comes from behind while kneeling slightly. He grasps her legs from the ankle lifting them a little off the ground as he penetrates from behind.

The "**eagle**" is a position in which the female lies on her back and lifts her legs while her feet are pointed towards the ceiling. She then spreads her legs as wide apart as comfortable while her partner kneels with knees spread for penetration. The male partner can hold on to her legs for support and to penetrate deeper.

The "**side saddle**" is a position in which the man lies back on the bed with his head propped up on a pillow and legs outstretched. The female partner crouches in a squatting position on his lap keeping her feet at his right thigh. After penetration, she leans back while placing her hands on the bed beside his left thigh. She uses her arms for balance and her legs to move her hips up and down while he keeps using his free hands for a little play.

The "**sphinx**" is a position. She bends one leg up, pulling her knee towards her body. The other leg remains stretched out. Her partner approaches from behind, placing one hand on either side of her hips.

The "**slide**" is a position in which the male partner lies flat on his back with his legs stretched out and thighs pressed together. The female partner lies on top of him with her legs stretched out over his. For enjoying a deep penetration, she can wrap her hands around his neck and slide her body up and down.

The "**Hollywood**" is a position in which the male and female face each other directly. While his back leans on the wall for support, he bends down and lifts her up to get into a standing sexual position. After the penetration is done, she presses her feet against the wall while he lies back onto the wall. With this, he supports her body weight by placing his hands under her bottom.

The "**tominagi**" is a position in which the female's head is propped up on a pillow while she lies on her back. She pulls her knees towards her chest while her partner approaches her on his knees and places her feet on his chest. After that, he grabs her knees for leverage while penetrating. During this, he can also lift her legs a little to change the angle of penetration and enhance the enjoyment.

The "**slip**" is a position in which the female lies on her back, head on a pillow but back flat on the bed. She bends her knees and pulls her legs up, spreading the legs enough to allow her partner to approach from the front. He slides in between her legs as she lifts her bottom allowing his knees to slide under.

The "**kneel**" is a position in which the male and female partner faces each other, both on their knees. His thighs are pressed together so she can straddle him for penetration. She can hold on to his neck for support, and he can wrap his arms around her waist to pull her close and support some of her weight.

The "**fold**" is a position in which the female lies on her back on the ground. While bending her knees slightly, she spreads her legs wide. The male sits down on the bed with his legs outstretched. He slowly slides his legs on either side of her body while pulling his whole body between her thighs. She needs to lift her feet a little off the ground during the time he takes to position himself in the correct spot. As he bends forward, she lifts her bottom to allow penetration while her partner wraps his arms around her midsection.

The "**spider**" is a position in which the male sits on the bed with his legs stretched out. The female partner sits on his lap in a position which allows the penis to penetrate. One of her legs is placed on either side of his chest to make the female feel comfortable. She leans nearly all of her body weight back onto her hands, placed on either side of his legs.

The "**glowing triangle**" is a position in which the female lies down on her back with legs enough apart for her partner to nestle close to her body. He places his knees down on the bed, and his hands are on either side of his partner's head. The female partner then lifts her hips by pushing up with her feet.

The "**seduction**" is a gratifying position in which the female lies back on the bed with her feet tucked under her bottom. She places her hands above her head, and the male approaches the female from the top with his legs stretched out straight. He holds his body weight on his forearms, which are placed on the bed.

The "**squat**" is a position in which the female stands on a low table. She stands facing away from her partner, who's standing on the floor. He approaches her from behind but stops just short of penetration. She squats down to sit on his penis. In this position, the male partner must be able to support his partner's weight by placing his hands under her bottom.

The "**Super 8**" is a position in which the female lies back on the bed with legs spread just far enough to allow her partner for penetration. Her feet remain on the bed during the Super 8. The male comes on top of his partner while holding his weight comfortably on his outstretched arms. For enjoying maximum pleasure, the female lifts her hips to meet the flow of the male partner.

The "**frog**" is a position in which the male sits on the corner of the bed while the female squats down in front with her back towards his face. He penetrates from behind while she controls the rhythm and depth of penetration. In order to reduce any kind of strain on the muscles of the female partner, the male places his hands on his partner's hips.

The "**shoulder stand**" is a position in which the female lies on her back on the floor. While placing her arms on the floor, she presses up and lifts her legs towards the ceiling. On his knees, the male partner grabs her bottom and enters from behind. In this position, the weight of the female partner should be centered on her upper shoulders. Due to this, it's called the shoulder stand position. In case the female requires help, the male can pull up on her bottom slightly to shift her weight to her shoulders.

The "**seated ball**" is a position in which the male sits on the bed. The female sits on his lap with her back towards his chest. Penetration occurs from this position. The male lifts his knees slightly, grabs on to his partner's midsection and curls over as he pulls her in towards him. During this, the female can move a little forward and hold her partner's feet or legs for getting the optimal support required for performing this step.

The "**suspended scissors**" is a position in which the female lies down on the bed. In fact, only the lower portion of her body remains on the bed while her left arm is suspended in air. The male then enters through her legs while straddling them closest to the floor. He holds on to her other leg with one arm and her midsection with the other, creating the scissor position.

The "**toad**" is a position in which the female lies on the bed with her knees pulled in towards her chest and legs spread far apart. Her body looks like a toad in a sitting position. Her partner lies down on top of her and places his arms around her neck to pull her close towards him. He penetrates from the front while she places her feet on the back of his legs just below his bottom to help in a deeper level of enjoyment.

The "**hinge**" is a position in which the female in on all fours, but her weight is on her forearms rather than her hands. Her legs are spread apart side. Her partner approaches from behind on his knees. One knee slide between her legs and the other is outstretched. She is in control of movement with the Hinge. She moves forward and backward, shifting her weight to rock the position after penetration.

The "**Stairmaster**" is a position in which the female partner squats down slightly on one stair, leans forward placing her knees on the next stair up and finishes the kneel by placing her hands on the next stair. He comes from behind while placing his knees on the stairs where her feet are located. He grabs her hips, enters from behind and uses the hip hold as leverage.

The "**galley**" is a position in which the male is sitting on the bed. His legs are stretched out straight, and the female straddles his hips and her bottom faces his chest. In this position, she uses her upper arms to support her weight. Then, she slowly moves her bottom back and down, allowing the penis to penetrate. She controls movement, rhythm and depth. His hands are completely free to massage and explore her body.

The "**fan**" is a position in which both the male and female stand upright while the female's back faces his front side. The female bends over a small table or chair while supporting her weight with the help of her forearms. The male approaches from behind, grabs onto her hips and does the penetration. In this position, all the movements are controlled by the male while giving good penetration depth, speed, and rhythm.

Kama Sutra Erotic Massage

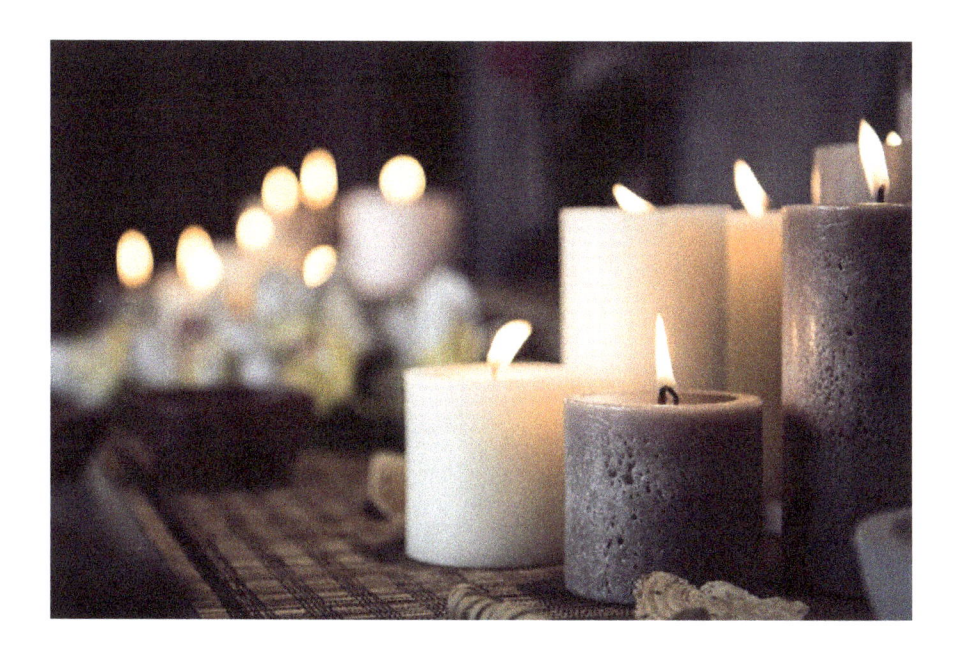

The Kama Sutra talks about massages and the best places to give massages. Some massages will lead to sex and some will not. A massage can also be a relaxing gesture of love for your partner, who is spending time with you at the end of the day. If you have massage oil, this will be a great addition, but if not, that's okay too. Use something like lotion to lubricate your hands and avoid skin to skin friction. Warm your hands before you start so that it makes them feel nice and doesn't send a chill down their spine when you first make contact.

When they are lying in a comfortable position, and you have lubricated your hands, begin to massage them gently. The touch of a massage gives a person a sense of being cared for, and it is even better from the person they love. A massage is a great way to show your partner that you care about making them feel good. After you have massaged their upper body or their feet, begin kissing their body where you just massaged it and then progress to kissing them on the lips. You can gradually move into touching each other's genitals or massaging them there. This is when it becomes an erotic massage. you can give a woman or a man to lead them to immense pleasure and enjoy a very sensual experience with them. An erotic massage is a way to show love to a partner, a way to be sexually intimate together and a way to make a person feel great without having a penis and vagina meet. Knowing these techniques is great for anyone who is looking to try new ways of pleasuring your partner in the bedroom.

Tips to Give an Erotic Massage to Him

A sort of erotic massage that you can try giving to a male partner is the prostate massage. As you know now, the prostate is a small gland located inside a man's body between the base of his penis and his anus. It is accessed through the anus. This type of massage is similar to anal play, but it is not the same, as the goals are different and so is the technique. The reason why it is better to give a man an erotic message here instead of on his penis is that he will be able to last much longer without reaching orgasm.

Performing this type of massage requires lots of lube for maximum comfortability. Once your fingers are well-lubricated, you can slide a finger or two inside of the man's anus very slowly. You will have to go slow so as not to shock the anus into closing tightly. You will need to work your way in gradually. Once in, you will be able to find the prostate by feeling around on the upper (front) wall of the rectum for a small lump that is rough in texture a few inches deep. Once you have found it, you can begin to gently massage it. You can move your fingers in circles and apply light pressure to it. This massage has the potential to feel quite pleasurable for the man. Communicate while the massage is occurring in order to give him the most pleasure possible.

You can perform this type of massage in a number of different positions. The man could by lying down while you straddle his legs, he could be on his hands and knees while you sit or kneel behind him, he could lie across your lap while you sit on a bed, or you could do any position that is comfortable for you.

This massage does not need to lead to orgasm; at least that is not the goal. If it happens, that is fine; however, the aim of this massage is just to provide a relaxing and pleasurable experience for him.

Tips to Give an Erotic Massage to Her

Next is the erotic massage for a woman. This massage involves the entire vaginal area, which is called the vulva. A Yoni Massage is a vaginal massage that is intended to open up the woman to her sexuality, her pleasure, and her sexual desires. As a partner, you can perform this type of massage for your woman to unlock her repressed sexual energy and help her to get in touch with it.

This can be done in a variety of ways, but the position we are going to discuss is a hot water Yoni Massage. Begin by setting the ambiance, either in the bathroom with a bathtub, or around your jacuzzi. Set up some candles, some flowers, or anything that will make the surroundings relaxing and calm. Begin by having her breathe deeply and focus on her body and its sensations. You can get into the water with her for added intimacy. Begin by slowly and gently massaging around her entire vulva and her clitoral area. The key to this type of massage is to do everything very slowly. Begin to massage her clitoris slowly and not with the intention of making her come. When ready, and with lots of waterproof lube, slide one finger inside of her vagina and gently begin massaging the upper wall. Here is where her G-spot is located. Encourage her to express and release any sounds she naturally makes. Move your finger in a circular motion slowly and with your other hand, massage her pelvic area and clitoris. This connects the inner with the outer. Continue to do this and let the experience unfold with no end goal in mind. If she reaches orgasm, she can do so, but if she doesn't, she can just enjoy the pleasures that she is getting from your massage. This massage is intended to reconnect a woman with her pleasure and allow her to focus on herself and her body.

After this massage, she will feel more in touch with her body, and if penetrative sex ensues, both of you will feel even more pleasure and intensity of orgasms because of how engorged and activated her vagina and clitoris will be.

How to Prepare the Body

Kama Sutra requires some flexibility and creativity to get all the various positions and movements right. In addition to what you will do physically, you also need to be in the right state of mind. As you anticipate the tantalizing pleasure that is to come, you need to prepare your body. Preparing the body is all about foreplay, to ensure that there is stimulation so that the explosive power of love making can occur. The process of preparing the body will awaken all the senses and ensure that the body is ready for full gratification.

Begin with the mind and the senses

For you to experience heightened intimacy and a connection with your partner, you need to stimulate the mind before anything else. This starts by the way that you set the scene. Your environment should be relaxed, and the way that it is arranged should be appealing for making love. Make an effort to decorate the room that you are in,

Have fragrant flowers around the room, so that their natural and delicate scent can fill the room. If you want to accentuate these scents even further, you can do so by burning aromatic oils. Remember, you are on the journey of arousal and you want that journey to be smooth so that when you reach your anticipation peak, you can join your bodies in magical movement. When you are preparing your body for a sexual encounter, you have a natural scent that should serve as stimulating. It is this scent that also draws you to your partner.

Starting with the mind enables you to ignite the passion of the one that you love. This requires you to stimulate the senses. Start with the sense of smell. Soak your body in a long warm bath that contains aromatic oils that appeal to your lover. In addition to smelling amazing, these oils will help to soften the skin considerably. As much as it is important to do what you like, this process goes two ways so make the effort to do something for your lover, by choosing a scent they prefer, and they will do the same thing for you.

Many times, people forget one essential part of the body when considering the sense of smell, and that is the smell of the mouth. You should pay special attention to your oral hygiene, as you will be using your mouth in kissing and embracing. This means that you need to have items that perfume the mouth, including light spices or a delicate mint. Whatever you use should be subtle and help keep your mouth fresh and clean smelling.

Next, focus on your sense of touch. As a woman, now is the time that you put on something that will glide over your body. Choose soft material like silk or satin and ensure that it allows for easy access to your intimate areas. Men can do the same, wearing silky boxers that accentuate the curves, bumps and shape of their intimate area. In addition to that delicate sense of touch, you also want to have a feast for the eyes. Your arousal will deepen when you see the effect that you have on your partner, so as a woman, your lover should be able to see your nipples harden and point and a man should be able to give a hint of the strength of his erection.

When your skin is against that of your lover, there should be no evidence of body hair as this will take away from the pleasure. Both women and men should shave their body hair at least every five days, particularly at the armpits and pubic area, and for men, they should also be clean shaven.

To add to this sense is the temperature of the room. It should be nice and warm, not hot or cold. If you are experiencing cold weather, make an extra effort to warm the room and in the heat, you need to have a window open to let natural air in and out. Avoid using a fan or air conditioner as this will affect the calm and sound in the room. You can further add to the sense of touch by using soft sheets and sprinkling flower petals all over them.

Now comes your sense of hearing. Have some tantric music playing in the background, with sounds that encourage you to make slow sensual movements so that you can glide in a gentle rhythm with your partner. To keep this mood going you must have no distractions, so switch of all your electronic devices. These include mobile phones, the television, beepers, tablets and so on. Unplug what needs to be unplugged, and even when it comes to lighting, choose candles and their soft light instead of a bulb – even a dimmed one.

The final sense is that of taste, and here you can have some delicious foods that will add to the stimulating nature of your lovemaking preparation. You cannot go wrong with fresh juicy ripe strawberries with whipped cream and champagne. Also add a light meal that you can easily eat with your hands and feed each other. When you are preparing to make love, you should not overeat or drink too much as this will dull your senses and take away from the experience that you are trying to create. Eat your food slowly and take time to chew everything sensually. As you feed your lover, give them small bits to eat and watch their mouth move and their eyes as well as you enjoy your meal.

You need to keep the mood up by talking to each other about anything that you consider romantic. This could mean that you are telling your lover how you feel about them, and that you are willing to trust them with your mind, body and soul. Look back at other stimulating moments that you have had so that the erotic memories can run wild in their minds, and their anticipation can pique as they think about what is coming up.

Finding Tantric Hot Spots

The next part of preparing for your love making is highly enjoyable, as it includes mapping out exactly what you are willing to try with your partner so that you can both reach heights of pleasure. There are a large variety of sexual positions that are illustrated in the book, and all of these will stimulate you in different ways. What you need to do is decide which of the positions that you are willing to try for during your love making session. Thinking about these will further stimulate your mind as you look forward to the pleasure that you are about to experience. In addition, this also helps to elevate the sexual energy between you, as when you are making live, you need this energy to be heightened so that all of your senses are at high alert. This will make it much easier to reach your climax.

A large number of the positions in the book are designed to fulfill a woman and give her pleasure by reaching her hot spots. There are positions which will help to tighten the vagina ensuring that when the woman is at the point of orgasm, her muscles will tighten up and contract which will increase the intensity of the orgasm. These positions often require the woman to hold her legs tightly together so that the man is squeezed tightly while he is inside her.

There are other positions that leave the hands of the woman free, which enables her to reach down towards her clitoris while the man is penetrating her and deepen her stimulation. These positions often require minimal energy from the woman to stay in place, which then results in her being able to freely play with herself, as well as with her lover during the entire duration of intercourse.

Deep penetration positions make it possible for the penis of the man to reach the woman's elusive G-spot during penetration. This is one of the most powerful hot spots that are on a woman and are the ideal positions to try after hours of stimulating foreplay if you are looking to get a mind-blowing orgasm.

Embraces

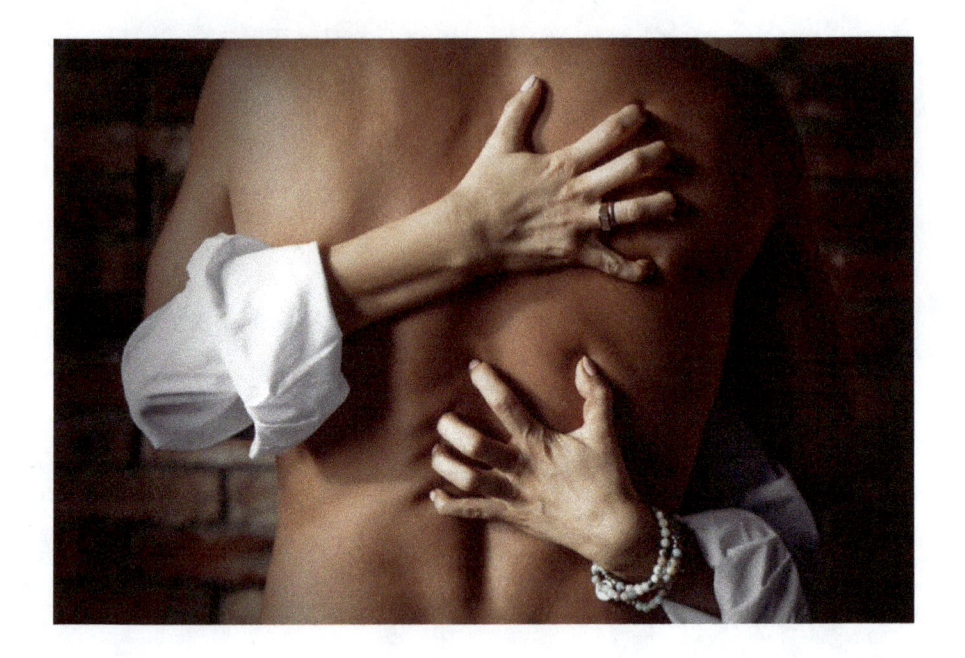

A large part of Kama Sutra techniques revolves around foreplay and getting the body ready for the pleasure that is to come. There are few actions that are as stimulating as an embrace, where to bodies come together, feeding off each other's warmth and experiencing the different textures and contours. The embrace is also referred to as Chatushshashti. You need to be able to explore the body of your lover so that you find those delicate areas and hot spots which will heighten the pleasure,

The typical embrace will mean that you are using more than just your arms. In Kama Sutra, you need to embrace using your entire body – a far cry from a hug. Starting at the top and moving down to the bottom of your feet, let your entire body come into contact with that of your lover, using smooth and circular movements that can best be described as a gentle caress. Alternate the pressure by touching some areas lightly and rubbing other areas with more intensity. You know the body of your lover, so by their reactions you will figure out which are the areas that you need to place your focus on. There is no right or wrong way to carry out an embrace, so you can choose to do it standing up or you could lie down and embrace while you are on the bed.

When you are embracing, remember that there is more to your body than just your hands. Use your hands as little as possible and instead take advantage of your cheeks and chest, your shoulders and even your thighs. The embrace should have gentle rubbing of your entire body for total stimulation. Also, your lips are a secret weapon, and you can kiss your lover gently, almost like you would imagine the flutter of a butterfly. The key is to take the process of embracing slowly and sensually.

Not all the embraces are considered equal ion Kama Sutra, as each one can bring out different feelings and pleasures. There are twelve in total, most of which you typically carry out naturally. Here are the embraces for you to try as part of your foreplay.

The Touching Embrace

This embrace normally takes place even before you have taken the time to set the mood and create a room which is designed to elevate your sensuality. This embrace is often unexpected, a soft touch that a man gives a woman to get her attention. There is so much a woman can read from this touch, as it can communicate affection, desire, love and lust. To prepare your partner for the final act of making love and intercourse, you should give them light touches for the entire day. This will have their minds racing, thinking about all the fantastic things that are to come. This is one of the first embraces that are ever done, typically before a couple have ever engaged in sexual intercourse.

The Forehead Embrace

This is an embrace that is all about intensity of feeling and the gentleness of a budding relationship. One of the lovers will use their mouths to plant gentle and light kisses on the other eyelids, mouth and forehead. This embrace ensures that there is close contact between the two lovers, and that they have the chance to look deep into each other's eyes from close range. It signifies the growth of a relationship, and that there is deep caring and affection. The gentle nature of this embrace can quickly stimulate a lover.

The Rubbing Embrace

This is an embrace that is done when two lovers have the opportunity to get close together when they are in a public place which happens to be a little lonely. Usually, they would be walking together with their hands intertwined and when they find a place where there is no one about, they would take the chance to rub their bodies against one another. This ensures that they can feel each other's contours and helps with their closeness as they look forward to going indoors and finding other ways that they can get close to each other.

The Twining of a Creeper

An embrace that is typically done by women, this embrace calls for the women to wrap herself around the man and cling to him using her arms and her legs. Their heads are bent towards each other as though they are about to kiss – but they do not. It is all about closeness and communicating love and possession through touch. There is also a sound that should be made with this embrace, the woman should gently say the words sut sut, as they have a way of increasing the intensity of the embrace. This embrace embodies affection and is deeply personal.

The Climbing Embrace

This is also referred to as the 'vrikshadhirudhaka.' Here is another embrace where the woman uses her legs to go around the body of the man. In this embrace, she will have one foot that is placed on her lover's foot, while her other foot is placed upon his thighs. To ensure she is balanced, one of her arms will go around the back of the man and the other arm shall hold on to the man's shoulders. While in this embrace, the woman will make some sounds that are similar to singing, or she will make a gentle cooing noise. She is supposed to appear as if she is reaching up to his face so that she can give him a kiss. It is the reaching upwards that gives this embrace its name.

The Pressing Embrace

Have you ever watched a love scene when one of the lovers gets pressed up against a wall, while the other users their body to press against them? This action is highly stimulating, as you feel the contours of your lover's body against yours, and often, can feel their heart racing on your chest. The pressing embrace is typically an embrace where you press your entire body against your partner, like a hug but with more intensity. This is a brilliant way for you to communicate the passion that you are feeling, and also to bring out the natural excitement in your bodies.

The Piercing Embrace

This is an embrace that is meant to tantalize a man, giving him a sample of what he can expect later during a period of lovemaking. For this embrace, a woman will find a quiet place where she is able to work on getting the full attention of the man. She will then bend forward before him, as if she is reaching to pick up something from the ground. While she is in this position, she will use her breasts and her nipples to 'pierce' a man by making a gentle movement that rubs against him. The main is them meant to take a hold of the breasts and gently fondle them. This is an embrace that is done before two people have become fully comfortable with each other.

The Milk and Water Embrace

This embrace is also referred to as 'kshiraniraka.' During foreplay, things can get so intense that you want to feel your partner inside of you if you are a woman, or you want penetration if you are a man. In the midst of all your kissing, you get into a position where you could experience intercourse, but your clothes are creating a barrier that stops it from happening. As your sexual organs rub against each other, you are stimulated, but have not yet given in to the temptation to start full intercourse. At this point, the foreplay has taken a turn that is highly erotic, and the embrace is highly passionate. In this embrace, the woman will typically be sitting on the man's lap, or they could be lying in bed with bodies rubbing against each other. It is meant to resemble a mixture of milk and water.

The Jaghana Embrace

To do this embrace you need to first identify the Jaghana. This is an area that can be found between the belly button and the thighs on a woman. To stimulate the woman during foreplay, this embrace requires the man to press this area using his own body, as though he is in a mounting motion. Then, he should gently scratch or bite her, while using his hands to hold onto her neck or her hair. The pain that results from this embrace should be very light and gentle, and this changes the pace of the entire period of foreplay, making it highly sensual. Gentle scratches along the back and arms are very erotic, and as long as there is no aggression, this can be the final embrace before moving into full intercourse.

The Sesamum Seed with Rice Embrace

This occurs when the woman and the man are lying together on a bed. They use their arms and legs to hold onto each other as tightly as possible, by ensuring that they are fully encircled. While they are in this embrace, their bodies shall rub together so that they can feel the strength of their arousal. This is an intense embrace which is often done at the end of the penetrative intercourse to reinforce the feeling of closeness in the afterglow.

The Thigh Embrace

This is an embrace that begins with a lack of consent, and ends with a transfer of power that is electric and stimulating A mar or a woman will be lying down on the bed and one of them shall forcibly press a thigh or both their thighs of their lover in between their own. Then they shall hold the position, so that they genitals are rubbing against the leg of their partners.

The Breast Embrace

This is an embrace that brings together the breasts of both the man and the woman. In this embrace the man will bring his breasts and then place it in between the breasts belonging to the woman that he wants to make love to. After he has placed it, he will press down on her, effectively rubbing against her to bring her stimulation to its peak.

Embraces often come quite naturally when you are looking for closeness for your partner, so although these embraces are considered to be essential for Kama Sutra, that should not stop you from having any other embraces which are natural to you. All that is important at the end of it is that there is passion in the embrace so that the resulting intercourse can be fruitful.

Love and the Kama Sutra

When it comes to love, there is much that can be said on how to obtain it, maintain it, and nourish it. While sex and love do not always go hand in hand, the Kama Sutra does emphasize the importance of love and goes to great lengths in order to detail exactly how a person can find love and then how they should go about ensuring that it lasts for a lifetime. Love begins with oneself, and only then can it be extended beyond that and onto someone else. That is why the Kama Sutra makes sure to include ways to enhance your own inner love and desire but focusing on self-care and self-adornment. The more you love yourself the more you can love others, and the more they can love you in return. If you are down on yourself, lack self-worth, or generally feel unlovable, then you will project that onto everyone that you come in contact with. You need to be able to present the best version of yourself possible, and always remember, there is nothing sexier in life than confidence!

Love is an extremely complex concept, and while we all may feel we understand what love is, if you ask 100 individuals to define love you will end up with 100 different responses. Love is defined as the feeling of attraction and desire that one feels towards another, but if you have ever been in love you will know that it extends far beyond that shallow explanation. Love and lust can often be confused with one another, since both play on attraction and desire, but the simplest way to break the two apart is to see love as something that is long-term, whereas lust oftentimes will fade or develop into love. When it comes to love, there are many factors that go into both falling in love, as well as staying in love with someone. Love is not easy, nor is it free from work, and in order to maintain a healthy, loving relationship you must be willing to sacrifice, compromise, and put in effort daily. Love is something that can grow and deepen with time, like a tree grows its roots down into the earth. What begins as only a small sapling can eventually turn into a mighty oak that even the worst of storms cannot damage. But how does one grow that tree of love? And how does one nurture it so that it is not cut down with time?

What the Kama Sutra Says About Love

The Kama Sutra discusses love in-depth and focuses heavily on marriages as the best type of union. With that said, however, it does acknowledge that not all sexual relations happen within the confines of marriage, and it does discuss the varying types of relationships that can occur. It is understood that love can strike at any time, with any person, and whether you are married to that individual or not does not always matter. That is why the Kama Sutra ensures that all aspects of love are covered so that it can be applicable to all situations and types of individuals.

One part of the Kama Sutra that is important to take note of, is the fact that the author makes sure to point out that love alone is not enough to sustain a relationship, nor is it enough to make a person happy within their life. While love is an important part of pleasure and being satisfied, it cannot be the only thing that you rely on in order to make you happy. If you pin all of your hopes and expectations onto one person, you are going to find yourself let down and dissatisfied, as one person cannot possibly meet all of your needs and desires. Instead, you should look at love as one piece of the puzzle that is fitted with other aspects in order to create a beautiful image.

From a historical perspective, the concept of monogamy was not as enforced as it is in today's society, and instead, there were many courtesans, or prostitutes, that were utilized without judgment. The Kama Sutra makes many notes towards courtesans, as their role in providing the ultimate sexual pleasure was very important even though it may not have involved love. Since this isn't as applicable in today's world, however, we can adapt these teachings as more of a personal guide on how to behave. The reason why courtesans were so desirable is because they were generous lovers who focused on their partner's pleasure and had qualities about that that made them engaging and entertaining. While you should never be something you are not just to please someone else, the idea of working on your own personality and qualities to enhance them and make yourself more interesting is certainly not a negative. We should all work towards building up who we are, being confident in ourselves, and feeling free enough to express our innermost desires.

Physical Attraction and Love

Although love requires much more than a simple physical attraction, the way a person looks is oftentimes the first thing that draws us to them. When you are looking to meet someone, and you know nothing about them as a person, you are going solely off of how they look to you. If someone is physically unattractive in your eyes, there is very little chance that you will want to pursue something intimate with them and thus the road to love is cut short.

The Kama Sutra acknowledges this and spends a lot of time discussing how to make yourself more physically desirable so that you can ultimately find love. We are in no way suggesting that your appearance is the only thing about you that matters, but we are saying that you should pamper and care for yourself in order to be the best version of yourself that you can be. From good hygiene practices to wearing your favorite sexy dress, making yourself look good will also make you feel good and that creates an energy that will draw someone to you.

Different Types of Love

The Kama Sutra breaks down four different types of love, which are:

- Continual Habit
- Imagination
- Belief
- Perception of External Objects

These four types of love are not necessarily limited to just within a relationship, and they can be extended to other aspects of life as well. Below will we break down these different forms of love, discuss how they relate to your personal love life, and even give advice on how to create, maintain, and nourish each type.

Love by Continual Habit

Love by continual habit is described in the Kama Sutra as the love that comes from repetition and practice of an act. In a non-romantic way, this is the love that may develop for a certain hobby as you continue to practice it and get better at it. The more you engage yourself and learn, the more you develop a love and passion. In a romantic way, this is the love that develops over long periods of time with an individual, either within or outside of a romantic relationship. For example, some people may begin as friends long before they become lovers. Over time, as they do activities together, engage in long, deep talks, and grow as people they eventually fall in love. This is the continual habit of being around someone and continuing to learn about them and grow together as a couple. This is a very strong form of love, as there is a great foundation to it, and it is built not on lust but completely on love. This is also part of what forms the love between two individuals who have been together for many years. Over the years that initial sexual attraction may begin to fade, and the lust that drew you together will start to become more of a slow-burning flame that keeps you both going. It is at this point that continual habit starts to strengthen and create the love between two people, as you live together and work together you practice the art of being in love. Falling in love is not the end, it is only the beginning, and over the years you will need to continuously work on that love and nurture it so that it continues to grow. Like blowing life into a fire, you are responsible for ensuring that the flame does not burn out.

Love by continual habit should also be extended to the individual, separate from any type of relationship. You should continuously work on learning to love yourself, showering yourself with affection, and strengthening those emotions within yourself. Make yourself into the partner that you so desire, so that whether or not you find that person, you already know you have that completely on your own. If you can meet your own needs, satisfy yourself, and be happy when alone, then a partner is simply the icing on the cake instead of the entire cake itself. This goes a long way in later creating healthy relationships with healthy boundaries because instead of feeling dependent on another person, you can simply enjoy being with them.

So, how do you create, maintain, and nourish love by continual habit?

- Actively spend time with the person you love or want to be in love with
- Practice being emotionally vulnerable with your partner
- Frequently touch your partner each day
- Take time each day to look in the mirror and appreciate something about yourself
- Share and create memories together
- Develop an idea of the future that you both would like to work towards
- Engage in sex frequently

These are only a very few of the ways in which you can create love via continual habit, and how you choose to do so is a completely personal choice. What is important is not how you do it, but more so doing it in a way that creates happiness and joy in both you and your partner. It is about building and growing together and working at love every day through the practice of making it into a habit.

Love by Imagination

Love by imagination is in complete contrast to love by continual habit, as it is far from physical and exists purely within the mind. This is the type of love that has no bearing in the real world, and instead is created within a fantasy of your choosing. An innate type of love, it is one that already exists within you and requires no effort or forming of habits in order to induce. It is a type of love that exists before your partner and will continue to exist despite your partner as it is not created by them. It can, however, be influenced and informed by your partner, but for the most part, it is simply an innate feeling that you have.

To break this down in more practical terms, we can start by looking at this love in non-romantic ways. Love by imagination is the way you love scary movies, or your love for dogs over cats. It's your love for sweet treats, spicy foods, or taking walks in nature. It's the love you feel when you think about your favorite book or movie, or when you ponder your future and all the things you will accomplish. As you can see, this type of love requires no effort and does not exist because you have worked on it. Instead, it is a love that is easy, effortless, and oftentimes cannot be changed. You can, however, alter this type of love as you age and grow, and different experiences will shape and guide our love by imagination. When you are young you may hate spicy foods, but as your taste buds mature you then find yourself with a passion for the heat. This requires no effort on your part; however, it does change and grow over time.

In a romantic sense, this is the type of love that exists even before you find your partner. Your personal preference in appearance, your desire for someone funny or smart, your different viewpoints and religions and all those other points that you think of in your head are all part of your imagination. If you close your eyes and visualize your ideal partner, you have love by imagination. Now, this type of love helps guide us towards the correct person for us, but it can also be a hindrance to finding a partner. In some ways, when you fall in love with the idea of someone, you set yourself up for failure. No person is perfect, and there is no one on the planet that will check every box or meet every criterion when it comes to your imaginative person. It is very important that you remember this, as those who seek to find perfection will instead only find loneliness. What you should do is use that love by imagination to guide you towards someone, without the expectation that they will live up to every item on the list. When you use love by imagination to guide you, you go into the relationship with a base of love already there. You know that you love people who have a great sense of humor, so you end up already loving that about your partner. If you know that you love someone who is fiercely intelligent, find a partner who is, and you will truly love that about them.

So, what are some ways in which you can create this type of love and maintain it in the long-term?

- Take the time to get inside your own head and find the qualities that are more important to you
- Always remember that no one is perfect, and find perfection within the imperfections
- Seek out people who match your own morals and standards

- Engage in activities you have a pre-existing love for
- Try out new things to find other activities you love
- Nurture your own interests
- Make meditation a part of your daily routine

Remember, this type of love is innate and is not something you can create over time. Take this as more of a starter love, one which draws you to someone and begins that relationship, rather than something used to maintain it over time. While finding someone with the right qualities will help ensure that you remain attracted long-term, it cannot sustain itself unless you strengthen and deepen that love in other ways as well.

Love from Belief

Love from belief is a love that is understood by both parties and is something felt deep within us. It is the type of love in which we have no questions, no doubts, and no fears. When we truly believe in love, when we believe in our feelings, we know that it is true and real. This is one of the strongest forms of love and it is the one in which meaningful relationships are built upon. Love from belief stems from great communication, high levels of trust, and mutual understanding that you both have developed with time and care. It stems from years of work, as well as effort and actions purposely used to create it.

When we discuss love from belief in a non-romantic setting, we refer to things like the love a parent feels for a child, or the love a person feels for a pet. It can also include the love you feel towards your personal accomplishments or achievements, as well as the love that exists within someone's religious beliefs. When you can feel an unwavering love and devotion, then you know you have love from belief. You are certain and sure of that love, there is no question in your mind that it is real and that you are secure within.

For romantic relationships, this is the love that lasts a lifetime. When you and your partner can look into each other's eyes and see nothing buy love reflected back, then you know that you have love from belief. You both believe to your very core that you love the other person and that they love you in return. You are certain that they have no malicious intent, that their reasons are pure, and that their heartbeats only for you. If you are fully your partners, and they are fully yours, then you are experiencing this form of love and you will feel safe and at home within it. But this love is not without work and effort, and in order to develop it, you need to both prove your trustworthiness, and have it proven to you by your spouse. High levels of communication are required so that you are both on the same page and there are no doubts or questions left between you. Trust must be both created and never broken, for if it is ever to be broken then love by belief will cease to exist.

Sacred Sexual Role of Women

In all ancient cultures, there were similar traditions, the essence of which was that a woman became a priestess of dedicating a man into the mysteries of love and sex. Egypt, Greece, Arabia, India, Tibet, and China - all of these countries, all of these unique highly developed ancient civilizations, shared this view. In ancient cultures, a woman was the epitome of sensuality and the guardian of creation, as had the gift of nature.

The role of women is multifaceted: a woman bears and nourishes every human being who comes into this world; she is the epitome of sensual beauty and eroticism.

Nine months we spend in the womb, eating, and evolving due to its vitality, gradually acquiring the internal organs and feelings coming through from her nutritious juices. We are like the fruit matures in the womb of a woman. As we age, we are born. Going out into the world through the mother's Yoni, we get the first sexual experience, which prepares us and still in pain, and the pleasures of this life.

The fact that all the people ever born were born from the womb of a woman made feminine nature magical and sacred. Sami woman's genitals were seen as an object of worship and called the Gate of Life, from which came to all living things.

Every man seeks to re-enter this realm of femininity through sexual contact.

Tantric and Taoist mystical teachings exalt exalting the human spirit is the power of the great Goddess, the divine principle of intuitive wisdom. The feminine energy, called Shakti, is present in every woman and man, as in all objects, living and non-living. Symbolized by a female form of the great Goddess has different names - Isis, the High Priestess, the Divine Mother, Kali, inner woman, the soul, or just Compassionate Home. This force, revered and extolled or causing fear and trembling, recognized in all ancient cultures of the world.

The ideals of female beauty are present in the Hindu writings such as the Kama Sutra and Ananga ranga. In them are various types of men and women following their physical, emotional, and mental characteristics.

"Nayika Sadhanatika" states: "A woman with whom a man will desire to do the art of love, to be exquisite beauty, her mind and body should be equally perfect. The sudden appearance of it will open the gates of emotions and capture the spirit. "

Another poetic text says: "A woman should be in the prime of youth, her eyes have to shoot arrows of love, features should express all that is good. On her lips - the nectar, the body resembles a graceful vine, and she must be in bright silk ".

In Chinese tradition, women also store and transmit the secrets of sex. Taoism refers to three different archetypal mentors in sex - Virgin Road, Maiden Dark Maiden, and elected. The most detailed Chinese erotic manuals, such as the classic "Secret Methods of Our Way," "Sexual Virgin Darkness leadership," and "Sexual recipes Virgin Road," written in the form of an intimate dialogue in which she devotes a man into the mysteries of sex.

Regarding the choice of women, which can be as a magical, dominant sexual partner and mentor, Taoist treatise "Secret Methods of Virgin Road" points out: "A woman is by nature gentle and soft? Her hair is smooth as silk, skin like velvet, bone-thin, it is not too small, and the growth is not high, not too thin and not thick. Her lips must be complete, and the Grotto of Pleasure, by nature, moist. During intercourse, she should spew copious liquid and move the body so that the man remains continuously agitated. The ideal age of a woman is between twenty-five and thirty years. "

The famous Indian text "Hevajra Tantra" speaks about the highest purpose of women as follows: "Those who are well-mastered Yoga should render the most excellent homage to his mother and sister, as well as dancers and laundresses, the same women from lower castes and of the noble rank. It should invest its efforts in Scepter Lotus Women's Wisdom. In this ritual, he achieves liberation. "

This enigmatic statement indicates the magical power of women. Later in the same text, we find the following explanation: "Higher knowledge is called" mother "because she gives birth to the whole world. Also, it called "sister," as her affection for a man is constant, "dancer" for her grace, fluidity, "laundress," because it gives the pristine freshness of colors everything it touches with his own hands. "

Initiatory role of women is enormous. When she takes an active role and explores the full range of the mysteries of sex during sex, it can give your lover incredible magical power. This power, the highest form of the Goddess Shakti, is a direct expression that reveals intuition, wisdom, energy, spontaneity, and playfulness of women who can sweep away all barriers. A woman should confidently devote her lover in the sexual sacrament. Success depends on the sincerity in relationships, the ability to trust and obey the higher ideals, from a sincere desire to give your lover something unique. Self-confidence and mystic power are the fundamental components of all initiation rituals. It is the Goddess within every woman who performs these rituals.

"The woman gives us the dedication through the same Yoni, from which the first man was born, - says one of the Tantric writings. - The woman devotes the same breasts that sucked the man when he was still a child. The woman devotes the same mouth that gently calms and lulls the man when he was just born. The woman - a high priestess of Tantra. "

Women in many ancient cultures often become temple dancers. The image of the dancer is closely associated with sexual energy and female dedicating force. "Dancing virgin has the power to start the process of sexual update", - stated in the Tantric tradition. In many temples of the ancient world were the dancers, whose sensual, self-forgetfulness, ecstatic dances passed the deep essence of eroticism.

The presence in the temples of India dancers shocked and offended by the British colonialists, who, in obedience to his Puritan morality, enacted laws to prohibit such activities. Sexual and sensual art of temple dancers forced the British to confuse them with prostitutes.

Temple dancers or Devadasi (literal servant of God) divided India into different categories. High Priestess were experts in various types of Yoga, and many years of training have mastered control of their bodily functions. They were mentors of Tantric Yoga and thus played a critical role. Their spouses thought of the temple of the Gods. It was believed that the welfare of the country depends on the rituals of the temple dancers.

One of the European researchers, Allen Ross brilliantly described the sexual role of an Indian temple dancer:

"Quiet entered barefoot girl. She knelt in front of me on my knees and kissed my feet. She was about thirty years old, and she was terrific. Her face was both feminine and childish. Her body was completely enveloped in a transparent gold silk sari. Arms, legs, and head are bare; they jingled gold jewelry when she moved.

Here she began to dance without any accompaniment. Sexuality was every bend plump lips Devadasi, every gesture of her arms, how she moved her head and stamped her foot in her views. Her nostrils widened and narrowed. Elastic, flexible body sensually bent, and it was a stunner.

I feel the electric charge of the erotic magic of this woman, and it seemed to me that it uses only a small portion of its magical features. Her dance, slow and ecstatic, was showing different sexual moods - from the charm of seduction, the excitation for master. Perhaps it lasted for hours, but I stopped for a time because I was utterly absorbed by the woman and watched her, unable to tear eyes. After that, she took possession of me. The strip was not, it is easy as a lizard, he slipped out of his clothes, and I saw the slender body of wild cinnamon. She told me to lie down on the carpet, and then there were only my lingam and Yoni in her cosmic union. She grabbed me, and I was obsessed with it.

She was one of those whom the Hindus call "women, splitting the nuts" because its sphincter muscles possessed fantastic strength. I just went crazy from what she was doing to me. She was making all the time whispering and humming sounds that immersed me in a trance. And suddenly, I felt my brain exploded, and I was in another dimension. Around were flashes of light and fantastic colors. The walls seemed to be melted, and I felt the divine ecstasy of every cell in your body. "

This description of a witness, or rather, the man who had sexual contact with a servant of the church dancing, allows us to judge that the power possessed by the dancer reliably.

This temple dancer must learn to control those reactions of the body, which are generally considered automatic. This reaction, such as breathing, to maintain equilibrium and emotions. This control is similar to that which is necessary in order to learn the teachings of Tantra. Emotions - the master key. Deliberately arousing emotions and spending, you can achieve personal liberation and pass it to another person. Sexual feelings very quickly can be called dancing. When the body is in order, the health and well-adjusted, the dance can actually be a great way of liberation.

Without a doubt, dancing in public and dance alone has an entirely different potential. This art can be practiced alone and for the partner. You can also improvise with a partner. Let your doubts and uncertainty will go away. Enjoy your creativity and spontaneity of their feelings.

The dance can express and give the person a lot. Dancing can be a means of communication, health exercise, or ritual of seduction and courtship. Of all the world sixty-four arts, says

Kama Sutra dance closest to the art of love. Dance woman has a unique potential to ignite the vitality of man and restore his lost strength. Musical rhythms of erotic dance will help to strengthen and maintain the intensity of love.

In many ancient civilizations of the world, there was also a tradition that some young virgin had become priestesses of love. It was honorable and even a sacred duty: those virgins, who were appointed to this role, considered themselves to be the chosen one of the Gods.

We know one of the earliest Greek myths. This myth tells of the origin of the Gods and explains how the God of time Chronos, who was the youngest son of Heaven and Earth, jealous of his mother to his father. He hid in an ambush and cut off insurgent phallus (male sexual organ) Sky with a sickle at the time when his father was making love with his mother. Phallus Sky Fell to Earth, and a few drops remaining in it, the seed fell into the ocean. From the seafoam, which is noisy and vigorously splashed on the shore, he was born a beautiful Aphrodite, the ancient Greek Goddess of love and feminine beauty.

Aphrodite, which was the water, became the wife of the God of fire Hephaestus. Although Hephaestus was the son of Zeus, the supreme God of the Greek pantheon, and pagan ruler of the world, he was born lame and ugly. Most of the time spent in the forge of Hephaestus, forging of gold and other precious metals, beautiful weapons, and beautiful decorations. Aphrodite was soon bored with her ugly and enthusiastic blacksmith craft husband. She was not satisfied with her husband sexually and therefore chose her lover Ares, a beautiful but ferocious, cruel mind and the recent God of War. When Aphrodite's husband learned of her infidelity, he set a trap. He forged in the smithy of a gold chain and caught her naked in the arms of a lover. Then he called to witness all the other Gods. Burning with shame, Aphrodite took refuge on the island of Cyprus, where he gave birth to Ares Eros, God of love.

Each of the ancient peoples had their Goddess of love and sex. Greek Goddess of love Aphrodite has many faces. She meets and Inanna - Sumerian Goddess of fertility, and Astarte - Phoenician Goddess of love, and Ishtar - Babylonian Goddess of love, and Isis - High Priestess and the Mother Goddess of the ancient Egyptians.

The cult of Aphrodite is widely spread in Cyprus and has had a significant impact on the entire Western mysticism. Thousands of people come to the island of Aphrodite from all over the ancient world to bow to her. In the temples of Aphrodite in Cyprus, where women must be given to anyone, you meet at its request. Only performing this rite of worship and service to Aphrodite, women received the right to marry. Money that in this woman was, she treasured as a talisman. This amount, as a rule, was purely symbolic: a young virgin had to surrender to a foreign traveler and small copper coins. The woman who served Aphrodite could not refuse intercourse with an ugly and weak man, a monster, who has a disability.

If from these unions' children were born, they gave to the temple of Aphrodite. A curious fact is that after such a ritual act of prostitution of women are still considered a virgin, and the children born of such a ritual act, called the birth virgin.

As we can see, the concept of the "birth of a virgin," "virgin birth" is the central concept of Christianity, it does not appear to Christianity, but there was already a few centuries earlier in Greece, Egypt, India, and other ancient civilizations. The dual role of the virgin prostitute had an impact on women's sexual psychology of the ancient world and affected the collective unconscious of women.

Erotic fantasies so many contemporary Western women somehow reduced to the fact that they imagine themselves as prostitutes, horny women who allow themselves to everything that could not afford actually to be decent women. In the other women of the same morbid interest is virginity. Soul shatter Western women between the archetypes, and pure evil woman is a relatively common cause of sexual neurosis in both men and women. The Europeans have accepted that a virgin pure, chaste, inaccessible, untouchable outside traditional marriage and fulfilled spiritually. Whore is rude, nasty and does not deserve respect. This idea of a highly simplified and schematic and have very little to do with the living reality. Sexual freedom woman and her selfless willingness to give their love to all men, in that love to the needy, do not exclude the spiritual and moral purity. Is the desire to donate his body crippled freak and utterly devoid of the joys of sensual love, a real example of supreme sacrifice, and thus the spiritual power of women? And at the same time, the so-called decent and chaste woman is often capable of quite cynically to figure out how she would "sell high," has entered into a valid marriage with the most financially wealthy man.

In the Eastern tradition, there is a specific definition - eternally chaste harlot. This definition perfectly conveys the complexity of a living woman's soul, the psychology of women, the duality of feminine nature and purpose. Meanwhile, simplified and schematic representations of female purity and depravity still filled with Western culture, despite the movement toward sexual freedom.

Since ancient times, a woman associated with the Moon because of its monthly cycle. A man associated with the sun and the elements of fire. Aphrodite - the embodiment of sensual beauty was born from the water and was married to the God of light. This is an example of this versatility symbolism. The relationship of the sun and the Moon are developed and perfected in the practice of sexual Yoga, Taoist Tantric tradition.

Western medieval art often depicts the Virgin Mary seated on the month, as on a throne. The Greeks had a triad of Goddesses virgins - Artemis, Hestia, and Athena. The symbol of the first of them was the Moon, and it is closely linked with Selene, Goddess of the Moon. Virgin Goddesses or Priestess in the Roman tradition were called at the beginning and the end of the ritual sacrifices. It was believed that they - the living embodiment of the Gnosis, the wisdom. They had to follow the sacred fire. One of the three Goddesses, Hestia, always depicted with a veil on the forehead with his right hand resting on the hip. Right hand resting on the bone - a typical gesture of the temple, sacred prostitutes, which is still considered an erotic, sexually arousing. It came from the depths of our collective unconscious.

Babylonian Ishtar, the Goddess of love and is usually depicted wearing a veil. It is believed that the mask hides its secrets from the uninitiated. The cover in ancient times was the traditional sign of virgins and prostitutes. Ishtar was the Mother Goddess; she had children. The rites of Ishtar to be treated like a harlot with a capital letter. Similar concepts are found in India, China, and other countries around the world, and they are always associated with the lunar mother who, although she was a virgin, she gave birth to children.

Practicing Love Making for A Healthy Body and Mind

The purpose of the Kama Sutra is not simply to guide the masses on different sexual techniques, but it is instead designed to promote healthy relationships and constructively use sexual energy. Unfortunately, several Western and Indian authors and interpreters have paid attention only to the sexual and physicality aspects of the book which has often led to the scripture's misrepresentation, as well as prevented the true meaning and benefits of the Kama Sutra from being experienced by everyone. The Kama Sutra has been a debatable topic amongst masses. The importance of this is it revolves around the true essence of a partnership between a man and a woman. Relationships are considered sacred; a man and a woman connect with each other to fulfill and satisfy their needs. When two people bond and meet their other halves, it is inevitable for them to oversee their partner's desires. Every emotionally healthy man and an emotionally healthy woman would want to please their partner until the highest degree. A sexual relationship is like constructing a building; unless the base is strong, the foundation cannot be powerful. In lovemaking, foreplay acts as the base of a sexual foundation followed by oral pleasure which towards the end boosts the intercourse portion.

It appears that the Kama Sutra, when well-practiced, can offer many health benefits for physical, physiological, and mental wellbeing. The reason for this is that many of the sexual positions listed have their roots in Yoga, and many of the benefits of Yoga positioning are mixed with lovemaking. Yoga is well known to have many benefits to the body, from flexibility and relaxation to increased blood flow and mental clarity. Combining yoga with intercourse is going to merge the benefits of both into one great experience. In fact, if you are considering taking up Kama Sutra as a part of your intimate life, taking up yoga would also be a good idea to help increase your flexibility. Because of these benefits, the Kama Sutra is widely considered a pleasurable way to stay fit.

As it has many health benefits, and similarly to tantric massage, the Kama Sutra is a practice that is being heavily promoted throughout the world and one being taught in many centers and institutions. Tantric massage is an erotic massage which encourages partners to get to know one another's bodies in order to learn what arouses their partner, outside of the typical arousal spots. Massage is a very important part of foreplay in the Kama Sutra, as we will cover later in this book. In addition, most relationship advisors encourage the use of techniques in the Kama Sutra as it establishes a very close relationship between the members of a couple. Also, such practice of the Kama Sutra promotes anti-aging, and it is said that simple practicing of the positions on a regular basis will cause you to stay forever beautiful. The reasoning behind this is the increase in blood circulation throughout the body, and the stimulation of muscles used to make each position during lovemaking.

The general purpose of this ancient text was not merely to educate masses about various sexual techniques, but instead to constructively use sexual energy and to promote healthy relationships between partners. The scripture has often been misrepresented with attention paid only to the sexual and physicality aspects, by commentators, authors, and interpreters. However, a deeper look reveals the Kama Sutra's teachings go far beyond just sex. The Kama Sutra encourages healthy relationships between partners, both in and out of the bedroom, and recognized the connection between the intimate parts of a relationship with the everyday motions.

The sex positions within the Kama Sutra have many benefits, well beyond just giving couples physical satisfaction. The range of sexual positions of the Kama Sutra has been found to give couples an extra level of satisfaction and also aid in the aversion of any physical, physiological, or psychological troubles. This works as the positions were designed keeping in mind the yoga positions and asanas (Sanskrit for the poses in a yoga exercise). Therefore, performing these positions helps to keep you healthy and fit. The sex positions in the Kama Sutra are said to bring get a man and woman relish their orgasms in the deepest and most intense ways. The best part is that the purpose of orgasm gets fulfilled in such a subtle manner that both the partners feel it as a part of the process. The pleasure level is so high that the orgasm becomes an integral part of it, and the maximum pleasure is actually derived with its combination.

When done correctly, Kama Sutra sex positions can bring not only physical pleasure but a source of bonding and curiosity between the individuals. Being able to find out what pleasures each other can be exciting and invigorating, enabling new feelings to emerge in the relationship. Sex has a positive impact on our mind and spirit and allows us to get to know ourselves better along with our significant other, almost as if taking a journey of self-discovery. The positions in the Kama Sutra, from the foreplay to the act of making love, encourage couples to be close and connected to one another. It is meant to allow couples to communicate with one another about what they like and what they don't like, as well as what they want to try in the future. Some of the advanced poses in the Kama Sutra also required the partners to trust one another for balance. All of these factors encourage a stronger relationship between two people. A simple touch, kiss or caress can rekindle old love or faded relationships. The Kama Sutra is an assorted series of texts that can ignite flames in new ways each time you make love to your partner. Considering the effects of the Kama Sutra, it can be called the Holy Book for Lovers looking forward to conquering love and create deeper affection amongst each other. The fact can't be denied that people sharing deep and purest form of sexual relationship enjoy closer understanding and intense bonds with each other which become inseparable with time.

Sex also aids in the stimulation of hormones such as oxytocin, which keeps you healthy and glowing. One hour of sex is the equivalent of a 15-minute jog every day and burns 200 calories per session. The practice of the Kama Sutra promotes numerous anti-aging properties in the body. One of the great benefits of the book is that it aids a couple in building a strong bond between partners, and also boosts beauty and vitality.

Those that have regular sex seem to be less burdened by arthritis or ailments of the heart. They are also said to live a long life compared to those who do not have sex on a frequent basis. Regular practice of the many unique positions will help keep you slim and toned with glowing skin and hair, and a sexy body. Sex also aids in the smooth flow of blood around the circulatory system, in turn promoting heart health. Stimulation of muscles during the action of lovemaking also helps to tone and sculpt the body. Making love with techniques with high and low intensities of burns as many calories as a person may burn while exercising. The major reason is because of the movements and heat the body creates which produce dampness and helps in developing physical fitness. Couples in modern age believe there are adverse effects of having sex which is gaining body fat, but as recorded in the Kama Sutra, a man and woman should equally participate in the activity which will involve both the parties actively indulging in physically satisfying their partner. The weight is gained by the women mainly when they don't show active participation during the process. It's also a proven scientific fact now that sex burns a high number of calories of a woman's body when she does the process properly and not only depends on the male partner for initiation and completion of the process.

Not only does sex have long-term effects, but the short-term effects can also be just as surprising. Sex can aid in fighting the stress of many forms: work, emotional, physical, and social. Regular sex also inhibits the release of vitamin D, which can have a positive impact on your skin, giving it a glow that would otherwise remain unseen. It is well known that because sex has such a powerful effect on your circulatory system, it aids in the prevention of certain cardiovascular and circulatory diseases.

Additional psychological effects can range from a reduction in anxiety, depression, stress, and enhanced self-esteem. Love making offers an enjoyable workout both on the inside and the outside of our bodies. Without sex, it can be difficult to find a generalized sense of wellbeing — especially for those individuals in relationships. A healthy intimate relationship between partners also fosters the partners to be closer to one another in other ways and increases the overall level of happiness and relationship satisfaction for the individuals in the relationship.

Couples having sex time and again have strong ties with each other compared to the ones who do not engage in sex often. With growing age, couples realize how sex played a pivotal role in keeping their bond intact. This increased divorce cases nowadays can be rightly blamed on the absence of devotion in the sex process. Yes, no doubt, there is a lot of sex between the couples, but it is done more for the purpose of satisfying one's lust than sincere love for each other. The Kama Sutra comprises of diverse basic and advanced techniques that can bring fresh excitement to your lovemaking each time you initiate it.

Potions and Sex Aids

The Kama Sutra outlined the best ways to attract your desired partner. If you tried all of the things listed in the Kama Sutra and still failed to attract the one you desired, the Kama Sutra outlined tonic medicines that were said to make a person more agreeable to that person.

Many of the things that are listed here are likely unavailable today and aren't as likely to be used in modern day society. The interesting thing about how these tonics were used when the Kama Sutra were written, is that even in modern day times we are still doing similar things to make ourselves more attractive to others, such as wearing makeup, changing hairstyles, and our clothing choices.

Since ancient times it is believed that drinking milk mixed with sugar and ghee before making love enhances the strength of a man, helps him perform better and sustain for a longer time while satisfying his woman. This is an old illustration from the Kama Sutra and is still followed by many in the modern age.

At the time of lovemaking, men and women are subconsciously under the pressure of pleasing their partners. It isn't very difficult for either of them to ejaculate quicker than the other. The concept of these increasing the sexual vigor of the man is the same as what we have today with the pills available to help a man be able to perform longer, as well as other sexual aids.

Another option is that if the man uses the same powder, mixed with the excrement of a monkey upon a maiden, she will not be given away in marriage to anyone else.

Obviously, the things they outline in the Kama Sutra aren't going to be used in modern times, and throwing monkey excrements at a woman is not going to get her to marry you, but that doesn't mean that the idea behind them is lost in history.

Today there are gels and creams and lubricants that are meant to make the acts of foreplay more enjoyable for both men and women. There are products that prolong the man's release, products that cause the woman's sensitive areas to swell and become more sensitive, and products that cause warming, cooling, or tingling sensations.

In the Kama Sutra text, there is also a reference to "Apadravyas." The Apadravyas is a piercing on the penis glan, the sensitive point at the end of a man's manhood, which passes through the glan vertically from either sideways or top to bottom. In recent times, piercing intimate areas of the body is not very popular. Moreover, it is a style whose significance is unknown and highly misinterpreted by many. In the ancient age, the act of piercing the hood of the penis was to intensify and stimulate a woman's deep-seated sexual spots. These are things that were put on or around the lingam to supplement its length or thickness so it would fit into the woman's yoni. Lingam also is known as Lingahas been associated with the Yoni since ancient times. Lingam symbolizes potential and energy of the Lord Shiva whereas Yoni exemplifies the womb and source of a woman. It is a symbol of Goddess that signifies strength and female creative energy. The coupling of the Yoni and the Lingam is epitomized as the unification of two bodies in one, an unresisting and submissive moment from which a man and woman can emanate another life that is a fusion of their own.

Vatsyayana said that these Apadravyas could be made of any material that suited the natural liking of the individual.

The Kama Sutra listed the following different kinds of Apadravyas:

The Armlet, or Valaya, was meant to be the same size as the lingam and had an outer surface made with rough globules.

The Couple, or Sanghati, is made of two Armlets.

The Bracelet or Chudaka, is made by joining three or more armlets until they cover the required length of the lingam.

Today, we have similar products on the market. The products that we have available today are often made of a soft silicone that is flexible and stretchy.

There were also options for women to use in the place of the lingam, or in addition to the lingam.

The Kantuka or Jalaka was a tube that was open at both ends, with a hole through it. It was outwardly rough and studded with soft globules. It was made to be tied around the waist of the woman and fit into the yoni.

When a Kantuka or Jalaka couldn't be obtained, there were other options. Some of these options were a tube made of the wood apple, a tubular stalk of the bottle gourd, or a reed made soft by using oils and extracts of plants. These were also tied to the waist of the woman.

These products likely remind you of some modern-day products that are available on the market. The items that we have available today are made from a variety of materials and in different shapes and sizes.

This goes to show that while the idea of sexual enhancements is more well-known than it used to be, it is by no means a modern-day idea.

Kama Sutra and Courtesans

At its core, the Kama Sutra is a book that is dedicated towards helping men and women who are in marriage understand each other much better and give each other the right amount of sensual and sexual pleasure. However, there is a core fact that this book acknowledges, and that is that it can get boring having only one partner for sex, especially for men. Therefore, there is some allowance for men to elevate their sexual pleasure by sleeping with other women.

When married, these other women are typically the wives of their friends. In case these types of women are not available, a man may seek to use the services of a courtesan.

Courtesans typically serve one purpose, and that is to help men get sexual pleasure and for offering this service, they are paid a fee for maintenance. It is possible for a courtesan to fall in love with the man that she has taken up with. When this is the case, her actions are quite natural. However, if she feels no love for him, then her actions are more forced. Even though they may be forced, she should behave as though she has love for him in order to gain his confidence.

To get the attention of the man, she needs to present herself in a certain way. To begin with, her dressing and the style she chooses is essentially. She should wear clothes that make her look good, and adorn her body with ornaments, though she must also ensure that she can expose some of her skin to gain attention. After all, she is expected to be standing by the side of the road attracting the attention of the people that are passing by.

Being a courtesan is riddled with hidden dangers, and she may be at risk of experiencing bullies or someone trying to steal with her. A successful courtesan will establish relationships with people who will help her maintain her activities. These friendships may be with people who are in law enforcement, like policemen and lawyers.

To help guide her decisions, she may seek the advice of astrologers, teachers of the 64 arts, or men who are learned. She will also need the council of powerful men to help her find her masters, as well as perfumers, vendors and so on. Even beggars can come to her aid when it is necessary.

The Type of Men for Courtesans

Considering that the courtesans who are skilled in Kama Sutra are determined to make money from their skills, there are certain types of men whom they pursue. These men fall into the following categories: -

- Young men who are virile and energetic

- Men who have an excellent source of income

- Men who are able to financially support themselves with no difficulty

- Men who have official and authoritative titles under the kind

- Men who think of themselves as handsome

- Men who enjoy giving themselves praise

- Men that are free from any relationship ties
- A man who may be a eunuch, yet wants to be identified as being a man
- Men who have income sources which are unfailing
- Men who naturally have a liberal stance
- A man who is proud of the fact that he is healthy
- Men who tend to be lucky
- Men who are recognized by other members within their cast
- Men who are only sons and come from families of great wealth
- A man who is brave
- A man who holds the position of the king's physician

Characteristics of a Courtesan

To appeal to the man and fulfill her purpose, the courtesan needs to have certain characteristics. These include the following: -

- A courtesan must be beautiful, and very pleasing to look at.

- The mannerisms of a courtesan must be gentle and amiable.

- She should also possess lucky body marks.

- The courtesan should be able to see the positivity in everyone.

- She needs to have an affinity for wealth, so that she can be motivated to provide the best possible offerings.

- She needs to enjoy sexual intercourse and be able to help the man attain sexual satisfaction.

- She should be sociable and able to interact well within social gatherings.

Courtesans are expected to go to a man who asks for them, but they should not do so immediately they have been asked for. This is because men do not appreciate things that come to them very easily, and in some cases, may even begin to despise her actions. Instead, she should not give her consent immediately, and rather wait to be asked for more than once. In her place, she can send singers or jesters to entertainment the man and find out what he is really feeling and thinking. This enables her to gather information on the man to determine whether going to him would be the right decision.

A man can start learning all about Kama Sutra by making use of the services that he can get from a courtesan. However, just like there are some women who may not have the required characteristics to become a courtesan, there are men who should not make use of courtesans. These men have the following attributes: -

- They may be unwell, or prone to catching certain sicknesses

- This man may have worms inside of his mouth, causing his breath to smell similar to human excrement

- The man may have a wife who he deeply cares about

- The man may be a thief

- A man who is proud and spends his time carrying out acts of sorcery

- A man who has no concept of what it means to respect another person or who communicates by being disrespectful

- A man who did not properly earn his money, or who uses his money to bring misfortune to other people

Courtesans who are like Wives

A man who has not yet married may have a courtesan who is living with him in the same way that a wife could. This should not be mistaken for an actual marriage as the courtesan is simply there to serve a purpose, and she is being compensated for her services.

While she is in this position, she needs to behave as though she were a wife, being chaste in her actions and keeping away from other men. In addition, her primary goal should be to ensure that the man is completely satisfied. In the Kama Sutra, respect is very important, and it links with giving pleasure. She should also keep in mind that she is there for the purpose of practice and keep herself from getting attached to the man. This is because there is every possibility that he will find a woman that he wants to marry, and when that happens, there will be no place for her in his home anymore.

To ensure that she is able to come off as a wife (even though she may not be one), she must know how to behave in every situation. First, she needs to have a much older woman who is dependent on her. This is so that she can ensure she continues to earn the money required, as her primary goal is to make money. This woman is key, as she will constantly be disapproving of the man, giving the impression that he is taking advantage of the woman and not paying enough. This is to keep him motivated and stop him from taking the courtesan for granted. The courtesan in turn needs to do whatever this woman tells her to do.

To gain the trust of the man, there are several things that the courtesan can do. She can start by putting him on a pedestal, always being wondrous when they are having intercourse, particularly about his prowess and knowledge of everything to do with sex. In addition, she should also relish in the different ways that he tries to pleasure her. She is to become his confidant, meaning that she should be able to keep his secrets and increase their level of intimacy by letting him know the things that she desires.

Courtesans are not meant to get angry with the men that they are trying to please, and in the event that they do, they need to be able to hide that anger effectively. They also need to do anything that the man wants during intercourse, taking guidance from him on where he wants to be touched, embraced and kissed and even expressing gentle care when the man is asleep.

She must take care of her personal hygiene, which is one way that she can reveal she cares for him without having to use any words to express her feelings. She must also be incredibly attentive, so that she can praise him when he speaks, laugh at any jokes that he makes, agree to dislike his enemies as much as he does, take care of him when he is unwell, and carry out all the other duties that would be expected from a wife.

How the Courtesan makes money

The courtesan is meant to help give the man the illusion that he is living with a woman as his wife, and therefore, the spell would be broken if she brazenly came to the man to ask for money when she wanted it. As a man, you would want to retain some of the sensuality and pleasure of having this woman who is willing to do anything for you. This limits the ways that a courtesan is able to get money, though, there are two major avenues that can be explored.

The first is by natural means which are lawful and accepted, and the second is by artifices. Courtesans do not have a fixed rate that they charge or expect. They get their pay based on what they believe the man is able to pay them, or to afford. Courtesans who want to get even more than this will make use of artifices, which means that the sole purpose of using this method would be for extortion.

There are various artifices that a man who has taken on a courtesan as a lover should look out for. To begin with, she may be bringing up numerous expenses that he has to meet on a regular basis, which need for him to instantly part with some money. These may include the need to make purchases for the home, including buying food to eat or drinks for refreshments. She may also want to retain her good looks by making use of clothes and perfumes. In looking for these funds, she will ask for more than she actually needs so that she can keep the balance.

Another artifice that can be used is praise. When men are flattered and told about how amazing and intelligent, they are, they puff up with pride, and are willing to make sacrifices to keep the praise coming. A courtesan will use praise when she wants to extort some money.

She may even come up with an excuse that she has been robbed while travelling to the home of her lover, the man, or after he has sent her to do something for him. If she claims to have lost jewelry, the man will feel compelled to purchase and replace it, or to give her money to find something new.

Should the direct approach prove to be ineffective, the courtesan can get other people to tell the man about the effort, time and money that she uses to see him and please him, so that he can then cover her expenses or debt.

In the Kama Sutra, men are encouraged to get wives, because wives are not taught to be deceitful for the purpose of exploiting their husbands. Instead, they are willing to work in partnership with them. This is different for a courtesan who may be willing to do and say whatever it takes to reach her final money attainment goal.

The Changing Lover

With time, the courtesan will begin to notice that the disposition of her lover towards her is changing, and she can identify this change if she notes the following behavior: -

- He begins to provide less and less for her, not meeting her needs as she has requested. This may also mean that when she asks to receive one thing, he gives her something else which she may not need.

- Rather than doing things or taking actions, he continues to give her promises for the purpose of keeping her hopes up. These promises never to materialize.

- He becomes dishonest, claiming that he is doing one thing, when in actual fact he is doing something that is entirely different.

- He starts to find other places to sleep and spends less time in his home. He will provide the reason that there is something that he needed to do for a friend.

- He begins to ignore her desires, especially during sexual intercourse.

- The conversations with his servants take on a mysterious air, and the courtesan is left out of the loop.

A courtesan needs to understand when these things are happening so that she is in a position to maximize on the money that she can receive as it becomes clear that he may move on from her soon. She should continue to treat him most respectfully so that he does not become aware of her intentions. This is particularly important if the lover is a man that is rich. Should he be a man that is destitute, she is free to leave him immediately, and behave as though they had never been together.

Kissing Techniques: The Kama Sutra's Subtle Forms of Sensuality

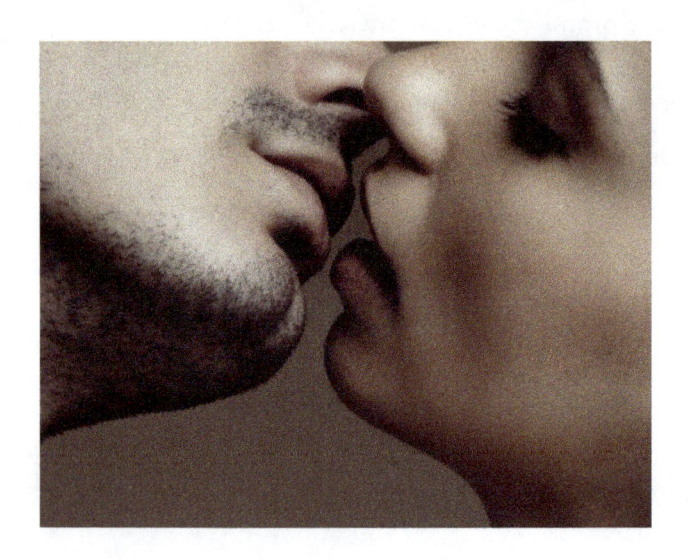

Listed within the Kama Sutra is an extensive range of kissing techniques which can be employed by lovers and those who wish simply to experiment with new forms of intimacy, both to inspire passion and fuel desire. Kissing is probably the biggest aspect of foreplay, and there are many different techniques that can be used when we are using our lips to communicate our level of desire with our partner.

Love cannot be verbalized which is why kissing and caressing is said to be a powerful act while having sex. There are more than 30 hot and affectionate moves for kissing your partner according to the Kama Sutra. Here's a list of the most passionate ones you must try,

10.) The Kiss to Distract: As the name suggests, this is a move made by a lover to seduce the other into lovemaking. You can move your mouth, kissing your partner on his eyes, ears, forehead, and cheeks. In this technique, you are not just bound to the face, but you can also move your way down, covering all parts of the neck, chest, shoulders and other raunchy areas that will spark a fire in your partner.

9.) The Kiss to Ignite Flames: This kiss is said to ignite flames as it covers the area of the mouth. It is a subtle approach to invite your partner that may seem impeccable but can erupt volcanoes of sexual desires in both the bodies. Scientifically, it is said that there are fine veins around the area of our mouths that are connected to the brain cells which create sexual tension within men and women.

8.) Contact Kiss: Similar to 'The Kiss to Ignite Flame', in this the male or female partners very softly and lightly move their lips over the others. Though this may seem like an innocent move, it can instigate exceptional thrills in lovemaking. One of the most irresistible moves inscribed in the book of love, Kama Sutra.

7.) The Throbbing Kiss: A series of kisses planted on a partner's mouth that is an embodiment of deep love and romance. This one has continued from the black and white age to an age of colorful visions with a magic unblemished and unbeaten.

6.) Clip Kiss: An uncommon practice among partners, this one involves licking the lips, gums and tongue jiggling. This move electrifies passion between the man and the woman.

5.) The Top Kiss: This one also known as 'Kiss of the Upper Lip' is a steamy encounter between lovers who love a little aggression during their lovemaking. A partner moves forward to softly bite the upper lip of the other wherein the other sucks the lower lip with the mouth.

4.) The Pressure Kiss: This is a level up in comparison with the one stated above, an audacious gesture by one of the partners which entails biting the lips and staying close to one another. This one needs to be done with sensitivity as could leave the lover with a swollen lip or mark.

3.) The Direct Kiss: This one could come off as one of the top-rated ones on the Kama Sutra kissing list. With a combination of kissing, licking and sucking while the couple looks at each other, this one evokes intense and irresistible desire within both the partners.

2.) Bent Kiss: This one is a great expression for a tall man or a woman sitting or standing in a position where she is a level above her man. In this move, one of them gently throws their head back while the other holds their chin and leans in for the kiss. A perfect one filled with emotions.

1.) The Askew Kiss: The most popular and a commonly chosen form of kissing by couples. In this one, both move their heads lightly kissing and pushing their tongues in each other's mouths. The latter makes it more compelling, one of the best ways to ignite love.

Kissing is a non-verbal act which speaks a million words. Each kissing move can high and low intensities on scales of innocence, passion, aggression, submission, dominance, and many other feelings that can bring lovers close within few seconds. A kiss can be a great way to welcome and bid farewell to loved ones.

A very important thing partners must understand while planting these kisses is that they can range from being subtle to aggressive. Unless both partners are not comfortable with the intensity and are on the same page, aggressive actions must be avoided by the couple. Biting of the lips or sucking on it can bring an evident swelling which could turn into a wound and would not look very pleasant outside the bedroom.

Some other forms of kissing are:

When we hold our lover's lips with two fingers, then touch those lips with our tongue, and finally, firmly press our lips to theirs, this is referred to as "The Greatly Pressed Kiss."

"The Kiss that Kindles Love" occurs when one looks at the sleeping face of their beloved and kisses the face to show intention or desire. While the lover may not be consciously aware of the kiss, it is thought that they will experience the kiss in their dreams and feel the desire of their partner. Unforeseen kisses can kindle love between partners. It is a spontaneous expression which substantiates immense longing in a relationship between a man and a woman.

"The Kiss that Turns Away" is another kiss often used in the movies, and it is performed in order to draw our lover's attention away from what they are focused on, or to detract from an argument. By forcing the kiss upon one's partner, one turns their attention to the kiss and their partner instead. The best kiss to make up to an angry partner. Kama Sutra is about reviving love between partners and building an unbreakable long-term bond.

"The Stirring Kiss" is a kiss that is said to arouse a man who is not in the mood for sex. This kiss is meant to be performed in a warm and seductive manner, not forcefully. This move lets a woman put forward her in-the-moment desire to have sexual pleasures. If a man is intrigued effectively, you may see him taking charge of the moment as if it were desired by him.

Finally, "The Kiss that Awakens," or The Sleeping Beauty Kiss, is one where we kiss our beloved while they sleep, perhaps when returning home late at night, and this kiss shows our love and desire. It is said that when performed correctly, this kind of kiss can wake even the soundest of sleepers and will most likely lead to further action.

Kissing is the first step to instigating fires within your partner, with that being said there are a few things you must take care of while initiating it,

Fresh Breath is a factor to be taken care of the most before getting into action. Chewing on gum or brushing your teeth could be great options for a good mouth odor.

Fragrance is an effortless way to attract your partner. As humans, we are sensitive towards enriching aroma. Adding a few tasteless drops of sensuous oils on your neck can ignite deep desires in your partner's heart.

Intensity must be communicated between kisses. Lovemaking is successful only when both the partners are satisfied and are equals. Enlightening a partner about the way each of you feels could make the process very smooth and easy.

While Vatsyayana described many different ways to kiss, he also warned that different people respond differently to kissing which plays an important role in any one's relationship. Kissing is the first step a couple takes toward a sexually active relationship, and a vital part of the couple's time together. If kissing is not being enjoyed by both partners, it can bring about an abrupt end to their relationship. There are various places where partners' plant kisses on each other which include kissing on the cheeks, forehead, neck and smooching which means kissing on the lips. It is an intimate and wordless expression of love that builds a strong and healthy relationship between two people. Kissing is also an essential part of foreplay and should not be overlooked when preparing for intercourse. Aside from actual penetration, kissing is one of the most personal and compassionate acts between a couple. Since kissing is such a huge part of the Kama Sutra, courting and foreplay, it is especially important to ensure that you are paying attention to your partner's cues when you kiss them, so you can determine what they do and don't enjoy when it comes to kissing.

When a man and a woman are romantically engaged with each other one of the first signs of approaching towards togetherness is moving in or hinting on kissing. Initially, one of the two partners or both can be hesitant, when one of them decides to take a step forward and makes an effort to understand the other person's desires the first kiss gets the ball rolling into the primary step of a relationship.

Vatsyayana also spoke of different types of games and teasing techniques, though he always cautioned against using teeth and hurting your other partner. Games can make lovemaking very exciting by playfully dodging the partner into making sexual moves or self-indulging yourself in an erotic act. Lips are one of the most sensitive parts of our body, being able to caress and speak to each other through touching of your lips can profoundly build the relationship. Due to the intimate nature of kissing, both parties involved are encouraged to be on the same wave of sexual energy to avoid the other from coming off as too aggressive. Softly nibbling or pressing your partner's lower lip between yours can add heat to the latter part of your love making. Brushing your partner's shoulders, moving your fingers down their spine, softly moving your fingers over their neck and edge of the lips can kindle carnal sensations in their bodies.

The Kama Sutra has a central agenda of turning sexuality into eroticism, and Vatsyayana wants us to realize that the unchecked ferocity of desire can overwhelm erotic pleasure, leading to a loss of humanity. What we once referred to as taboo 'perversions' is now considered regular fare on television and in movies, where small specific, specialized professions exist catering to the satisfaction of almost every sexual excess. Amongst this, the Kama Sutra's project to rescue the erotic from the raw sexual finds many supporters. The Kama Sutra is a classic in the world of literature, which infuses sexuality with playfulness, and proclaims an ethic of the erotic combining sensuality with senses. For couples who like exploring their wild side, the Kama Sutra is the best manual for rewarding their partners with immense pleasure and physical appreciation.

How to reach ecstasy in 10 difference position

A good puzzle can change the experience, and a considerable number of individuals pass up ground-breaking climaxes just by neglecting to analyze. Try not to resemble them. Utilize this straightforward manual for discovering a place that delights both you and your accomplice.

Stir Up Positions that Allow and Deny Eye Contact

The principal thing to note about sexual positions is that they are about considerably more than merely discovering approaches to enter your sweetheart all the more profoundly. How you position yourself when you have intercourse brings numerous different things into play. Yet, above all, you can either meet as you fuck or lose an eye to eye connection.

A decent method to begin is by picking a place that lets you investigate each other's eyes. Set up closeness, grin with your eyes, at that point, start moving onto more out of control, progressively athletic procedures. Eye to eye connection is the establishment stone after that; everything else gets constructed.

Switch back and forth Between Different Partners Being in Control lady and man finding their best sex position

Test in various rooms and places.

At the point when you begin to have intercourse, don't surrender it over to one accomplice to look after force. Positions like the preacher require the person to work more enthusiastically and cut-off the lady's degree to communicate. Blending it up with some time in the Cowgirl position can allow each accomplice to sparkle.

Trial with Standing Positions

Here's another unusual stunt that individuals overlook: Sex doesn't need to occur on the sheets of your bed either. Standing positions like the "Ballet performer" can permit speedier, more profound entrance.

You should simply stand, confronting one another. Presently, the female accomplice raises one of her legs as the male enters her straight away. It's speedy, essential, and extraordinary for quick ones.

Concoct a Sexual Feast in the Kitchen

Another good thought is to explore different avenues regarding various rooms of the house. For example, the kitchen is an incredible spot to expand your sexual skylines. The tallness of work surfaces and tables appears to have planned considering sex.

At the point when you're in the state of mind, put down your spatula, push away your plates and locate a little space to roost. The person should simply kill the gas and get the chance to work.

Do Some Stretches and Get Athletic?

If you've at any point watched pornography, you're presumably acquainted with a portion of the more genuinely requesting sex positions; however, have you at any point attempted them?

If not, here's the thing to recall positions like the Wheelbarrow are extraordinary enjoyment. However, they take quality and adaptability.

By all methods, attempt them, yet do a couple of stretches before you do as such, as no one needs to pull a muscle at the essential minute.

There's More than One Way to Come from Behind

For some individuals, sex from behind is about doggy-style, yet that is crazy. Doggy, for the most part, includes accepting a creeping position. However, you can likewise try different things with the Flatiron. Right now, lie face down with straight legs, at that point marginally raise their hips, making an erotically bent profile that folks can't help it. It's an incredible minor departure from a stale old position.

Make sure to Watch Your Speed and Power

At the point when you begin evaluating diverse sexual positions, recall that your accomplice will encounter new sensations. You may be entering her more profound than at any other time.

She may be arriving at climax all the more rapidly or encountering snugness. It could be awkward on the off chance that you push excessively hard and too quickly, so be mindful of what she says and locate the ideal musicality for each position.

Utilize Your Shoulders for Faster, More Efficient Orgasms

Sex is actually about climaxes, when you get down to it, however here's the entertaining thing: most folks have no idea which positions carry ladies to climax the quickest. One approach to do so is by working your shoulders into your daily sexual practice.

Attempt positions like The Fusion, which includes your accomplice, putting her legs on your shoulders. If she gets drained, you can change to The Spider, with her feet on the bed once more. It's an incredible method to make variety in the vibe of infiltration, which assists with making quicker, progressively energetic peaks.

Get Far Out with the Snow Angel

Some of the time, trying different things with sex positions can appear to be peculiar, yet don't accept that because a situation seems to be weird, it won't work. Take the Snow Angel, for instance.

Here, you lie looking in inverse ways, and the man infiltrates "backward" as the lady sees his rear end rising and falling. The opposite infiltration is an astonishing inclination, and there's consistently scope for a rim job if all works out positively.

Tight Positions Can Make Small Penises Seem Larger

Are you stressed over the size or length of your penis? Here's one extraordinary stunt to redress: Sex positions could be the appropriate response, not costly siphons or false pills.

Positions like the Flatiron or the Corkscrew that include the lady fixing her thighs together can compensate for littler enrichments by causing her vagina to appear to be more tightly.

Locate the Perfect Position for Oral Sex

Sex positions likewise aren't just about all out the sex. How you approach cunnilingus is additionally extremely significant.

Couple on the couch attempting another sex position

Try not to expect that because a situation appears to be unusual, it won't work!

Analysis, Experiment and Experiment Some More

No one should restrain their sexual coexistence to current positions. On the off chance that you do, you'll be scamming both yourself and your sweetheart.

The two people can draw in their curious minds and discover places that heighten their closeness, lead to increasingly pleasurable climaxes, and are inherently incredible enjoyment. So, don't be timid. You will love it.

How to use sex toys to your advantage and give yourself and your woman

I have been a fanatic of sex toys since the time I purchased my absolute first vibrator at the Condom world in Boston. My school beau and I were "on a break," and I thought the ideal approach to manage the vacancy was to purchase a vibrator and an extravagant shanty lunch for myself. At the point when I returned home soon after that, I opened the bundle, hurled in individual batteries, and had my psyche blown. There was no returning after that.

However, in those days, my fantastic vibrator wasn't something I talk. Unfortunately, my masturbation propensities, as well, I minded my own business. So even though I had this incredible toy that I cherished (it was child blue!) and from which I had some extreme climaxes, it was my mystery for quite a while. Also, the idea of utilizing it with my accomplice, once our "break" finish, was not feasible. I'm so cheerful I don't feel that way any longer.

One of the main reasons my sexual coexistence with my present accomplice is so acceptable is because we use sex toys. Neither one of us avoids acquainting new ones with our sexual exercises, nor do we both concur that variety in sex toys additionally upgrades our sexual encounters with one another. Nowadays, I can't envision having intercourse without them in our tool stash.

On the off chance that you still can't seem to utilize a sex toy with your accomplice, at that point, it's an ideal opportunity to shake things up. Here are ten extraordinary reasons why you ought to be working them into your sexual coexistence.

1.   They Take the Pressure Off of You

Now and again, it's challenging to climax — regardless of how giving your accomplice is. As per the Kinsey Institute, 70 percent of ladies need a type of clitoral incitement to accomplish climax. While instigation of the clit can achieve with fingers or the tongue, contingent upon your position, those probably won't be choices. In going after that additional assistance from a vibrator, you're removing the strain to climax from yourself, which can help open a wide range of ways to climaxing with your accomplice as a rule.

2.   They Take the Pressure off Your Partner

Regardless of to what extent you've been with your accomplice, they're never truly going to have the option to hit that detect how you can when you're stroking off. In bringing a sex toy or (at least two) to the room, you won't just ease the heat off of your attempting to accomplish climax, yet it will reduce the temperature of your accomplice, as well. Sex will be unwinding, and tingly, similar to it should be, for both of you.

3.   You're more likely to Have Multiple Orgasms

When you ease the heat off yourself and your accomplice, at that point, you can make way for climaxes that are simpler to reach, however, even different orgasms. It's a logical truth that vibrators improve sexual fulfillment. So among toys and your accomplice, you're setting yourself up for an extraordinary circumstance that will load with a more significant number of climaxes than you'd most likely get if it were merely you and your accomplice sans the battery-worked toys. It continues onward and proceeding to go.

4. Investigation Makes for Hotter Sex

Investigating new domains in your sexual relationship doesn't only open up ways to things you never realized you might appreciate; however, it makes a significantly more unique sexual bond. Let's face it: You always remember the primary individual who bound you to the bedpost.

There are remote control toys that your accomplice can control from over the room (or over the globe); butt plugs for those hoping to evaluate butt-centric play; dildos, which are extraordinary while a lady is accepting oral sex; and whips. Blindfolds, cuffs, choke ball, and areola braces for those hoping to take their BDSM game up a couple of indents.

5. They Encourage You to Try New Positions

With this investigation going on, you never know what kind of bent up positions in which you'll get yourself. The Kama Sutra may have just 64 seats, yet with enough inventiveness and a sex toy as your guide, you may discover there are more than that.

6. Common Masturbation Is Awesome

We realize that masturbation is great for you, but at the same time, it's sweltering to observe each other jerk off. Furthermore, it's incredibly instructive, as well.

Stroking off with sex toys before your accomplice not just gives them what you like and how you get yourself off. However, it's excellent foreplay. Men, mainly, are incredibly visual animals, so for them to be permitted behind the drapery to watch you stroke off necessarily causes them to feel like they've made it big. What's more, on the off chance that you're into somebody, at that point, you'll most likely be similarly into watching them joy themselves.

7.   They Can Help Bring Fantasies to Life

The chance that you've for the longest time been itching to play the definitive teacher, there's a whip for that. Or then again, perhaps you've been fantasizing about playing a cop and cuffing your accomplice to the bed — whatever the case might be, sprucing up, pretending, and utilizing toys as your props are the ideal approach to remove the dreams from your head and into this present reality.

8.   You'll Be Giving the Middle Finger to Any Stigma

Even though sex toy use is more typical than any time in recent memory, they still once in a while get negative criticism for being just for "desolate" ladies, and even a few men are scared by "contending" with sex toys. Truly, folks? By utilizing toys in the room, you and your accomplice will be giving the finger to those old legends — which just has sex considerably increasingly fun.

9.   You'll Finally Put Your Curiosity to Bed

In this way, you've been joyfully making the most of your sex toy solo, yet you've been pondering exactly how much satisfaction it would be on the off chance that you acquainted it with your accomplice. All things considered, what are you sitting tight for at that point? When you check out it, you can quit pondering, and begin having the best sex of your life.

10.   Getting Them Together Is a Bonding Experience

In buying sex toys together, you can choose which ones will be a solid match for the both of you. There's a colossal assortment of toys out there, and with a little experimentation, you'll see one that works for you two. Likewise, don't be reluctant to converse with the sales reps — they can lead you the correct way.

Step-By-Step Positions for The Beginner

Here, we are going to cover some positions that are great for beginners to Kama Sutra, step-by-step. As time has gone on, the names of the poses in the Kama Sutra have changed through translations and interpretations. We have tried to keep the names below as close to their original names found in the Kama Sutra as possible, but in some places that were not feasible due to translation.

Many of these positions weren't intended to be used from the beginning of intercourse through climax. Instead, it was encouraged that the partners use a variety of positions, since each position targets different sensitive areas for the woman, and this would ensure both partners reached the highest climax that was possible.

The positions below are some of the easier positions within the Kama Sutra. Although at first, they may seem a little confusing or complicated, we encourage you to give them a try a couple of times before you decide that you aren't capable of performing them effectively.

Widely Opened: This position isn't far off from the well-known missionary position, making it a good position to start with.

1. The woman begins by lying on her back on the bed. The man kneels on the bed. The woman raises her buttocks and thighs and wraps her legs around him.

2. The woman arches her back and leans backward as the man thrusts in and out of her while holding her underneath her back.

The Yawning Position: This position is a great position for beginners, as it is simple and easily varied to find the perfect angle for each partner.

1. The woman lies on her back and stretches her legs up and outward until they are totally extended and widespread in the air. The legs can be raised to the armpits of the man.

2. The man kneels and enters the woman while holding the woman's hands for support.

Indrani: This is similar to the missionary position, although it requires a little more flexibility on the part of the woman. If she can get into position, the lovemaking will be worth it.

1. The woman lies on her back with her knees bent up to her chest.

2. The man then kneels in front of the woman and enters her.

The Close-Up: This position is intended for snuggling. It is a very intimate position that allows for feeling your partners body all over in skin-to-skin intimacy.

1. The woman lies on her side on the bed while the man snuggles in behind her. The woman can feel him right up against her back.

2. The woman then spreads her legs and helps the man enter. He then draws his legs together and begins to thrust. At the same time, the woman closes her legs, holding him inside her.

The Rocking Horse: This is an innovative position that puts the body into unfamiliar postures, which allows for increased pleasure for both the man and the woman. Although this position will put you and your partner into an unfamiliar pose, it is not a difficult pose to achieve.

1. The man begins by sitting cross-legged on the bed. He supports himself with his arms behind him resting on the bed.

2. The woman then kneels on him and spreads her legs on either side of his pelvis, slowly lowering herself onto him.

3. The woman then holds the man close with their bodies touching. She will move up and down using her thigh muscles and a circular motion of her hips.

The Cross: Another variation of the missionary position, this position ensures deep penetrative lovemaking and gives the woman a higher level of stimulation.

1. The woman lies on her back with one leg extended and one leg bent while the man holds the bent leg.

2. The man rests on his knees and places his thigh over the woman's extended leg.

3. The woman then takes her bent leg and touches the backside of it to the chest of the man, with her leg straight up against the man.

The Glowing Juniper: This is a romantic position that allows the partners to look each other in the eye while they engage in intercourse.

1. The woman lies down on the bed on her back, with her legs outstretched and slightly spread apart.

2. The man slides between her legs leaving his legs outstretched as well.

3. The man wraps his hands around the woman's waist and lifts her slightly into position for penetration.

4. If the man is flexible enough, he can lean over the woman to kiss her belly, or he can simply hold her and look into her eyes.

The Prone Tiger: This is a fun position for couples to try if they are looking for something a little different to try.

1. The man sits on the bed or another hard surface with his legs outstretched.

2. The woman straddles his body with her back to his front.

3. She lowers herself onto his lingam from the straddling position.

4. Once the man has penetrated the woman, she stretches her legs out as straight as possible and grabs onto the man's feet for leverage.

The Triumph Arch: This is a position the combines the previous two positions into one that is a little trickier, but just as romantic as the Glowing Juniper.

1. The man sits on the bed, or another hard surface, with his legs stretched out in front of him.

2. The woman straddles his body, resting on her knees while she is facing him.

3. Once the man has successfully penetrated the woman, she leans backward and rests her head between the feet of the man.

4. Like in the Glowing Juniper, the man can now either lean forward to kiss the woman, although in this position he is in line with the breast, not the tummy, or the man can look into the woman's eyes.

The Magic Mountain: This position is a rear-entry position that doesn't require the woman to hold her weight up.

1. Make a mountain out of firm pillows. You want the mountain to be high enough so that when the woman is on her knees and leans over, her hips are at a right angle.

2. After the woman leans against the pillows, the man kneels behind her with his legs on the outside of hers. From this position he penetrates her.

The positions above are all relatively easy to achieve, although they may take some practice to get perfect. Each one of them is going to bring your lovemaking to a higher level than ever before. Not all of the above positions may be right for you and your partner, however, experimenting with them is half the fun. Once you have had fun with the above poses, if you are feeling more adventurous, read on to find some more challenging poses you and your partner can experiment with while lovemaking.

Advanced Love Makers

If you have mastered the beginner poses or see yourself as a more adventurous, flexible love-maker, than these advanced poses are probably just what you are looking for to add a little spice to the bedroom. Be aware that each of the following poses is probably going to take a little bit of practice before you begin to reap the reward of immense pleasure from them. Do not give up if the position you want to try does not work out for you the first time. Some of the positions are going to require a couple of attempts before you get them perfect without any difficulties. There is also going to be that feeling of awkwardness until you are comfortable with the position.

The Balancing Act: This pose is going to require that you can balance effectively in order to make the most of this position. It may seem complicated, but once you have achieved this position, it isn't as difficult as it sounds.

1. The man begins by lying down on his back with his legs wide enough to accommodate the woman.

2. The woman must now carefully sit in between the man's thighs.

3. The man then enters the woman by gripping her hips with the help of his thighs.

The Rowboat: This position is going to require complete synchronization between the man and the woman to achieve maximum pleasure.

1. To begin, the man and the woman sit facing one another with their legs spread. The woman's legs should be spread first with the man's legs on top of the woman's legs.

2. The man lifts his legs and hooks his knees into the woman's elbows. The woman then raises her legs up and hooks them into the man's elbows.

3. Both partners begin thrusting, moving forward and backward in equal frequency. This is where the name Rowboat comes from since both partners need to work together, much in the same way they would if they were to rowboat.

The G-Force: As the name implies, this position is a gravity defying position that is difficult to get into. Once you have gotten into the position, it is quite arousing and allows for incredibly deep penetration.

1. To begin, the woman lies down on her back and raises her legs up in the air and brings them close to her chest.

2. The man then kneels in front of her and, holding her ankles, brings her close to him. The man will start bending the female's ankles towards her head to raise her lower back off the surface.

3. Once the only parts of the woman touching the surface are her shoulders and her head, the man enters her from the top holding her ankles, with her legs touching his chest and resting on his shoulders.

4. The man remains in an upright position and thrusts downwards into the female.

The Deck Chair: This position is not nearly quite as complicated as some of the other positions. However, it can be a little tricky to figure out if you are a beginner.

1. The man is going to sit on the bed, or a hard surface with his legs stretched out in front of him. He is going to lean back with his elbows slightly bent.

2. The woman is going to lie between the man's legs with her head on a pillow. She is going to slowly inch her hips towards the man's hips while putting her ankles up on the man's shoulders.

3. Once the man has penetrated the woman, she can place her hands on his thighs to give herself leverage to maintain the thrusting action.

The Squat Balance: This position requires strength and skill on the part of the man, and balance on the part of the woman.

1. The woman is going to stand on a stool or the bed while the man is behind her.

2. He is going to place his hands on her bottom so that she can sit on him while she leans into his chest.

3. From there, he can penetrate her from behind while she holds onto his arms for support.

The Peg: This position may look as though it is going to be complicated to figure out. It can be difficult to get it started, but once you have it figured out, it's not very hard at all.

1. To begin, the man is going to lie on his side.

2. The woman is going to begin by lying curled up on her side with her head down towards the man's feet. Her knees need to be brought to her chest with the man's legs sandwiched between her thighs.

3. The woman is going to hold onto the man's legs while he guides her to him with his hands.

It is recommended that you take this position slow until you are sure that you and your partner are balanced and that no one is going to get hurt while in the position. Once you are confident with the positioning, you can pick up the pace.

The Suspended Scissors: This position is for those who are in very good physical shape. This position is going to require extreme physical fitness and flexibility. Ensure both partners are strong enough to perform this position. This position is going to be incredibly difficult to get into, but once you have mastered it, you are going to be addicted to it.

1. To begin with this position the man has to stand firm while holding the female by her waist to support her weight.

2. The woman puts one hand on the floor and holds the arm of the man with the other hand.

3. She now lifts one leg to the outside of the man's leg and brings her other leg up between the man's legs. The only part of the woman now touching the floor is her hand that she put on the floor in step two.

These are just a few of the sexual positions detailed in the scriptures of the Kama Sutra. I will leave the rest, for now, to your imagination and discover for yourself when you delve into the sensuous world of the ancient teachings in this mystical text, which has stood the test of time and is still revered as one of the great keys with which we can unlock our inner sexual prowess.

Conclusion

As you go on in your sexual life, stay open-minded, and never stop listening to your body. People change and you will likely change as well. By being open to these changes and being receptive to them in yourself and your long-term partner, you will be able to ensure you are always getting the most out of sex. Don't forget to communicate with your partners in order to better understand them and sex in general, as communication leads to learning and this is a great thing when it comes to sex.

The hope is that this book has given you the tools you need to keep your sex life fresh and ever-changing by introducing you to the world of Kama Sutra. Maybe you have tried some of the positions from the Kama Sutra before, and you needed help in order to learn more. Maybe you have tried all of the classics and are looking to get into something completely new and adventurous. Whatever experience you came with, I hope that you are leaving this book having learned a few new things to take with you into your sexual adventures from here forward. I hope this serves as a tool for you to explore and discover yourself and your future partners.

There is something for everyone in this book, so continue to pass it on to your friends and your partners so that we can live in a world of educated and informed sexual beings. The Kama Sutra is a guidebook for love, and everything involved in loving another person. It is more than just a book of sex positions, but these days most people only know it for its complex and flexibility-requiring positions for intercourse. The book of Kama Sutra includes a general guide to living well in ways other than through sex. It includes a guide to foreplay, a guide to kissing and touching, as well as other ways to achieve intimacy with your partner, such as bathing together and giving each other massages. I hope that after reading this book, you understand and can appreciate this text in a new way.

In addition to the positions enclosed in these pages, I hope that you learned how to focus on your pleasure and the pleasure of your partner, how to be present during sex, and how to become more sexually intuitive in order to feel the most pleasure possible. What a waste of pleasure it would be to always have sex in the same positions over and over and never fully reach your potential for orgasm! If you haven't already, try some of the things you've learned through reading this book, and I assure you that your sex life will be much better for it!

You are now ready to go off into the world of sexual exploration and have great orgasms from here on out. Stay curious and keep learning!

I hope this book was able to help you to understand the history and origin of Kama Sutra and how it relates to you and your relationship. Through this reading, I hope you are encouraged to discover what you find pleasurable in your life and relationships. After reading this book, I hope you are not only inspired to read more in depth on the topic but also excited about the prospects of self-discovery in the wake of lost pleasure.

Lovemaking, or sex, is an activity we will all participate in at some point in our lives. Knowing what we find pleasurable and what we desire to achieve during the course of the activity is key in having an enjoyable experience. When partnered with a significant other, discovering each other's body can be one of the most enjoyable parts of the experience. Kama Sutra in its entirety can help you understand and decipher your own desires and beliefs while also introducing you to an ancient culture that was historically known for their sexual beliefs and practices.

You were given advice on different biting, kissing, embracing, and foreplay techniques to help bring you and your significant other closer. This book was intended to provide you with a guided outline of historical Kama Sutra beliefs and the most popular practices and techniques. In order to obtain more information on the topic of Kama Sutra, further research can be done on one's own to learn more on the topic.

The next step is to either read more on Kama Sutra or recommend this book to a friend or family member. Sharing the knowledge of pleasure can be priceless in terms of wealth. Giving your family member the option of discovering themselves and their loved ones is a gift that would take centuries to match. Your next step could also be to approach your own significant other, if applicable, and perhaps experiment with some of the ideas in this generalized overview. Perhaps if some enjoyment is found, more research could be done on the topic to enhance your sexual activity and health even more.